ENDOCRINOLOGY RESEARCH AND CLINICAL DEVELOPMENTS

CYSTIC TUMORS OF THE PANCREAS

ENDOCRINOLOGY RESEARCH AND CLINICAL DEVELOPMENTS

Additional books in this series can be found on Nova's website under the Series tab.

Additional e-books in this series can be found on Nova's website under the eBooks tab.

ENDOCRINOLOGY RESEARCH AND CLINICAL DEVELOPMENTS

CYSTIC TUMORS OF THE PANCREAS

ROBERT GRÜTZMANN
EDITOR

nova biomedical
New York

Library of Congress Cataloging-in-Publication Data

ISBN: 978-1-53612-523-8
LCCN: 2017953951

Published by Nova Science Publishers, Inc. † New York

Contents

ACKNOWLEDGMENTS

A scientific book like this one can only arise through the laborious work and intensive research of many individuals. I would like to express my gratitude to all those researchers who invested countless hours in the multiplication of knowledge, eventually leading to this print.

I would like to thank all those who have worked on and helped with the completion of this book, especially my esteemed co-authors.

A special thanks goes to Dr. Maak for taking care of the necessary accompanying activities a work like this requires, namely planning, preparation, and communication with the co-authors.

Last and not least I want to thank our patients who taught us so much.

Robert Grützmann, MD, PhD, MBA
Professor of Surgery
Head of the Department
Department of Surgery

INTRODUCTION

Robert Grützmann, MD, PhD, MBA
Department of Surgery,
Friedrich-Alexander University Hospital Erlangen, Germany

Cystic tumors of the pancreas today are diagnosed more frequently in clinical practice, mainly due to an increased use of the modern advanced imaging modalities.

Bland cysts of the pancreas most often develop after chronic or acute inflammation of the pancreas. However, the current knowledge concerning the development of cystic neoplasias of the pancreas is still rudimentary.

Histopathologically, 90% of pancreatic cystic neoplasias are represented by four types: serous microcystic (SCN), mucinous cystic (MCN), intraductal papillary mucinous (IPMN) and solid pseudopapillary (SPN) neoplasias. Surgical treatment of these lesions can be highly challenging and occasionally demands complex surgical approaches that should be put in the hands of skilled pancreatic surgeons in experienced high-volume centers.

While some of the described cystic tumors are harmless, such as SCNs of the pancreas, others such as IPMN and MCN harbor relevant malignant potential. The differential diagnosis of these lesions is critical for the patient- but often difficult. In addition, surgical treatment, even in the hands of skilled surgeons in centers of pancreatic surgery, can be complicated and can result in relevant morbidity and mortality.

Therefore, it is of great importance for all doctors treating and advising patients with cystic tumors of the pancreas, i.e., surgeons, gastroenterologists, radiologists and pathologists as well as for the general practitioner, to have funded knowledge in regard to epidemiology, pathology, diagnostics and prognosis of the various pancreatic lesions, regardless of the necessity for surgical treatment.

Together with recognized specialists in this field from Europe, the United States, and Japan, the authors offer a broad and detailed overview over diagnosis and the current treatment strategies for patients with cystic tumors of the pancreas.

SECTION I. EPIDEMIOLOGY

In: Cystic Tumors of the Pancreas
Editor: Robert Grützmann
ISBN: 978-1-53612-523-8

Chapter 1

EPIDEMIOLOGY OF CYSTIC PANCREATIC TUMORS

Matthias Maak[1,*], MD, PhD and Robert Grützmann[1], MD, PhD, MBA
[1]Department of Surgery, University Hospital Erlangen, Friedrich-Alexander-University, Erlangen-Nuremberg, Erlangen, Germany

ABSTRACT

Cystic tumors of the pancreas were believed to be rather rare. The widespread availability and use of cross-sectional imaging with multidetector-row computed tomography (CT) or magnetic resonance imaging (MRI) allowed asymptomatic pancreatic cystic lesions and specifically neoplasms of the pancreas to be detected with increasing frequency. The prevalence of pancreatic cysts in the general population is described with 2.4% to 19.6%, making them a rather common incidental diagnosis. Cystic lesions in the pancreas consist in ~30% of injury- or inflammation related cysts like pseudocysts, paraduodenal wall cysts and

[*] Corresponding Author Email: Matthias.Maak@uk-erlangen.de.

infecion related cysts, ~60% are cystic tumors, the remaining lesions are congenital or miscellaneous cysts.

Pancreatic cystic tumors are categorized by the WHO in four subtypes, each subtype having a benign and maligne form: serous cystic neoplasms (SCN), mucinous cystic neoplasms (MCN), intraductal papillary mucinous neoplasms (IPMN), and solid pseudopapillary neoplasms (SPN).

Keywords: epidemiology, cystic tumors, pancreas, serous cystic neoplasms (SCN), mucinous cystic neoplasms (MCN), intraductal papillary mucinous neoplasms (IPMN), and solid pseudopapillary neoplasms (SPN)

INTRODUCTION

Cystic tumors of the pancreas are a realtively new topic in medicine. Until the end of the 1970s pancreatic cystic lesions were considered rare and mainly consisted of and were divided between serous and mucinous neoplasms of the pancreas [1-3].

The following decades showed a tremendous increase in the development and widespread use of new imaging techniques, leading hitherto to an increase in the number of diagnosed and resected cystic lesions [4, 5].

Consequently, new tumor entities were identified, described, and the knowledge about these tumors, their behavior, biology, morphology and pathogenesis advanced [6-9]. For example, it has been just about 30 years since intraductal papillary mucinous neoplasms (IPMNs) were introduced to medical vocabulary, and since then studies and knowledge about this entity flourished.

Before modern cross section imaging and its widespread availability, cystic tumors of the pancreas were considered rare and thought to cover only 10%-15% of all cystic lesions of the pancreas and 1%-5% of all pancreatic tumors [10, 11]. Nowadays it is known that this assessment underestimates the incidence of pancreatic cystic tumors.

Due to the widespread use of cross-sectional imaging with multidetector-row computed tomography (CT) or magnetic resonance imaging (MRI) nowadays, most asymptomatic pancreatic cystic lesions and specifically neoplasms of the pancreas are detected incidentally with increasing frequency [12-16]. The prevalence of pancreatic cysts in the general population is described with 2.4% to 19.6%, making them a rather common incidental diagnosis [13, 15, 17, 18]. Pancreatic cystic neoplasms themselves account for more than 50% of pancreatic cysts, even in patients with a history of pancreatitis [8, 12, 16, 19-21]. Although we would like to focus on cystic tumors of the pancreas, a short overview about cystic lesions of the pancreas helps to put the relative frequency in perspective.

Cystic Lesions of the Pancreas

Asymptomatic cystic lesions of the pancreas are detected in more than 2 percent of patients who undergo abdominal cross sectional imaging for unrelated reasons [8]. Table 1 shows the characteristics of studies focusing on the prevalence of pancreatic cysts. Those study results show a rather broad range.

In detail the study by de Jong et al. retrospectively analysed 2803 mostly asymptomatic patients with magnetic resonance imaging who underwent preventive screening at their own initiative and expense.

Table 1. Characteristics of studies on pancreatic cyst prevalence [8]

Study	Number of patients	Prevalence (%)	Technique	Patients with known pancreatic disease excluded
de Jong et al., 2010 [17]	2803	2.4	MRI	Yes
Laffan et al., 2008 [13, 19]	2832	2.6	CT	Yes
Lee et al., 2010 [18]	616	13.5	MRI	Yes
Spinelli et al., 2004 [16]	24039	1.2	MRI and CT	No
Zhang et al., 2002 [15]	1444	19.6	MRI	No
Kimura et.al., 1995 [22]	300	24.3	autopsy	No

Prevalence of cystic lesions was 2.4% and increasing with age [17]. The study by Laffan et al. retrospectively analysed 2832 consecutive computed tomography scans of the abdomen, excluding patients with known diseases or symptoms of th pancreas. Prevalence of cystic lesions was reported to be 2.6%, also increasing with age [13]. Lee et al. described an also age-depending prevalence of even 13.5% in a retrospective analysis of 616 MRI-scans of patients without pancreatic diseases. The relation of prevalence of pancreatic cysts in relation to increasing age is visualized in Figure 1 by de Jong et al. [8].

A prevalence of pancreatic cysts of 1.2% was described by Spinelli et al. in a retrospective computerized analysis of 24,039 MRI and CT scans in 2004 [16]. Of these 58%, meaning 0.7% of the total study population, did not have a history of pancreatitis. MRI scans of 1444 patients were reviewed by Zhang et al. leading to a prevalence of cystic lesions of the pancreas of 19.6%, but without exclusion of patients with a known history of pancreatic disease [15]. Kimura et al. performed 300 autopsies on elderly patients (>80% were older than 65 years) without exclusion of pancreatic diseases and described a prevalence of 24.3% of pancreatic cystic lesions. An explanation for the rather broad range of prevalence is the differing study designs. The selection of the study population, inclusion or exclusion of patients with pancreatic disease, and choice of the imaging modality, with each technique having its distinct sensitivity and specificity for detecting cysts [8].

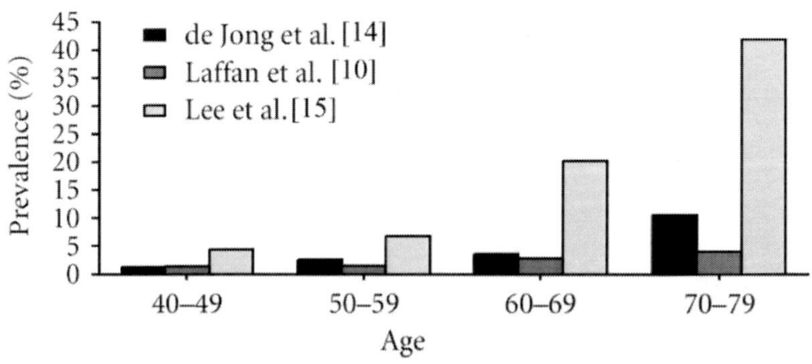

Figure 1. Prevalence of pancreatic cysts in relation to increasing age [8].

Table 2. Estimated relative frequency of cystic lesions of the pancreas [6]

Types of Cystic Lesions in the Pancreas

- Injury-related and inflammation-related cysts (30%)
  - Pseudocyst
  - Paraduodenal wall cyst
  - Infection-related cysts
- Neoplastic cysts (60%)
  - Ductal lineage
    - Mucinous type (30%)
      - Intraductal papillary mucinous neoplasm
      - Mucinous cystic neoplasm
      - Intraductal oncocytic papillary neoplasm
      - ''Retention cyst,'' ''mucocele,'' and ''mucinous nonneoplastic cyst''
      - Cystic change in ordinary ductal adenocarcinoma and other invasive carcinomas
    - Serous (clear-cell) type (20%)
      - Serous cystadenoma
      - Oligocystic (macrocystic) variant of serous cystadenoma
      - von Hippel-Lindau syndrome–associated pancreatic cysts
      - Serous cystadenocarcinoma
    - Not otherwise specified
      - Intraductal tubular carcinoma
  - Endocrine lineage (<5%)
    - Cystic pancreatic endocrine neoplasm
  - Acinar lineage (<1%)
    - Acinar cell cystadenoma (cystic acinar transformation)
    - Acinar cell cystadenocarcinoma
    - Cystic/Intraductal acinar cell carcinoma
  - Endothelial lineage (<1%)
    - Lymphangioma
  - Mesenchymal lineage (<1%)
  - Undetermined lineage (5%)
    - Solid-pseudopapillary neoplasm
  - Other
    - Mature cystic teratoma
- Congenital cysts (<1%)
  - Duplication (enterogenous) cysts
  - Duodenal diverticula
  - Others
- Miscellaneous cysts (<5%)
  - Lymphoepithelial cyst
  - Squamoid cyst of pancreatic ducts
  - Epidermoid cysts within intrapancreatic accessory spleen
  - Cystic hamartoma
  - Endometriotic cysts
  - Secondary tumors

Basturk et al. [6] provided a detailed overview of pancreatic cystic lesions and their estimated relative frequency in the experience of the authors as shown in Table 2. As described, the whole of cystic lesions in the pancreas consists in ca. 30% of the cases of injury- or inflammation related cysts like pseudocysts, paraduodenal wall cysts and infecion related cysts which we do not focus on any further. The majority of pancreatic (60%) cystic lesions are cystic neoplasms, the remaining lesions are congenital or miscellaneous cysts. These estimations were comfirmed by Valsangkar et al. in a analysis of 851 resected cystic tumors [23].

Using pathological terms, pancreatic cystic lesions can be classified into neoplastic cysts and non-neoplastic ones, which can be furtheron be divided histologically into epithelial cysts (retention cysts being the most common) and non-epithelial cysts (pseudocysts being most common) [24].

Cystic Tumors of the Pancreas

The World Health Organisation (WHO) categorizes pancreatic cystic tumors in four subtypes, each substype having a benign and maligne form: Serous cystic neoplasms (SCN, cystadenoma and cystadenocarcinoma), Mucinous cystic Neoplasms (MCN), Intraductal Papillary Mucinous Neoplasms (IPMN, IPM-adenoma and IPM -carcinoma) of the main and the branch duct type, and Solid pseudopapillary neoplasms (SPN, SP adenoma and carcinoma) [25, 26].

The key epidemiologic and biologic characteristics of pancreatic cystic tumors are summarized in Table 2 and are described in more detail in the following paragraphs.

Serous Cystic Neoplasms (SCN)

Patients with SNCs are predominantly (75%) elderly women with a median age of approximately 60 years [8, 27-30]. SCNs can arise anywhere in the pancreas [2, 31, 32] and can occasionally involve the entire organ. SCNs account for approximately 5-20% of resected cystic lesions of the pancreas and 16-39% of resected cystic tumors [9, 23].

A small number of cases of malignant serous cystadenocarcinomas have been described, but it is gererally believed that SCNs have very low malignant potential [33]. SCNs can be associated with von Hippel-Lindau disease [32, 34, 35].

Mucinous Cystic Neoplasms (MCN)

Patients with MCNs are almost exclusively (95%) perimenopausal women (mean age 48 years, range 16-84 years) [6, 36, 37], but less common in postmenopausal women than in women of childbearing age [38]. The tumors present mostly (95%) in the distal pancreas, i.e., body and tail [9, 36, 39], and do not communicate with the pancreatic duct [39].

MCNs account for 8-40 percent of cystic lesions of the pancreas and for 10-49% of neoplastic cystic lesions of the pancreas [9, 12, 23, 40]. The malignant potential of MCNs varys from 6-36% [36, 39, 41] with reports up to 50% [42].

Intraductal Papillary Mucinous Neoplasms (IPMN)

IPMNs are connected to the ductal system of the pancreas, they can involve the main pancreatic duct (main duct type, MD-IPMN), can be confined to the branch ducts (branch duct type, BD-IPMN), or can be a combination of these two (mixed type, MT-IPMN). Two third to seventy percent of IPMNs occur in the head of the pancreas [6, 43], predominantely the MD- and MT-IPMNs. BD-IPMNs are more likely to involve the uncinate process, have an equal sex distribution [44], and arise in younger patients [45-47]. MD- and MT-IPMNs occur more often in male patients. The mean age at time of diagnosis is 68 years, with a range of 25 to 94 years [44]. IPMNs account for 18-38% of cystic lesions of the pancreas [23] and for 21-33% of cystic neoplasms of the pancreas [12, 40].

The malignant potential of MD-IPMN is with 57-92% rather high whereas it is moderate to high 6-46% for BD-IPMNs [38].

Approximately 30% of patients with IPMN show synchronous or metachronous tumors in other organs like the stomach or colorectum [48, 49] and they have been reported to be associated with the Peutz-Jeghers syndrome [50] and familial adenomatous polyposis [51].

Solid Pseudopapillary Neoplasms (SPN)

SPNs are not considered true pancreatic cysts but rather to be degenerative necrotic changes with cavity formation [52].

It is condidered a rather rare tumor entity comprising 10-27% of all resected pancreatic cystic tumors and 4-21% of all pancreatic cystic lesions [53, 54]. SPNs predominantly occur in women in their twenties or thirties [53, 55, 56] and are located throughout the pancreas [9, 57] with a cumulation in tail or body [19]. SPNs have a relatively low malignant potential with reported incidence of malignant transformation of 15% [58].

Other rare cystic tumors of the pancreas are also reported in literature and although detailed data is scarce, their existence should be noted:

Cystic pancreatic endocrine neoplasm (CPEN) are rare and represent about 4-8% of resected cystic pancreatic tumors and 10-17% of resected pancreatic neuroendocrine tumors [59]. They occur equally in women and men, the predominant age is 60-70 years. CPENs can present anywhere in the pancreas. 25% of patients with CPENs have also MEN I syndrome [60].

Cystic degeneration of ductal adenocarcinoma and other solid tumors like endocrine tumors, have been described as very rare, representing less than 1% of cystic tumors[5]. They occur slightly more often in men, the age at diagnosis is 60-70 years.

Acinar cell cystadenomas and cystadenocarcinomas are rather uncommon, diagnosed more in men than women at the age of 40-70 years [61-63].

Table 3. Epidemiology and characteristics of cystic pancreatic tumors [5, 8, 9, 19-21]

Type	Sex distribution	Age (years)	% of pancreatic cystic lesions	% of cystic tumors	location in pancreas	malignant potential
SCN	F>M (75%/25%)	50-70	5-20	16-39	anywhere	very low
MCN	F>M (95%/5%)	40-60	8-40	10-49	body/tail (95%)	6-36%
MD-IPMN	F<M (40%/60)	60-70	18-38	21-33	head	57%-92%
BD-IPMN	F=M	50-70			head/ uncinate process	6-46%
SPN	F>M (90%/10%)	20-40	4-21	<10-27	body/tail	low
Cystic endocrine neoplasm	F=M	50-60	4-8	10-17	anywhere	variable
Ductal adenocarcinoma with cystic degeneration	F<M (slight)	60-70	na	<1	na	high
Acinar-cell cystadenocarcinoma	F<M	40-70	na	<1	na	high

REFERENCES

[1] Compagno, J., Oertel, J. E. Mucinous cystic neoplasms of the pancreas with overt and latent malignancy (cystadenocarcinoma and cystadenoma). A clinicopathologic study of 41 cases. *American journal of clinical pathology,* 1978; 69(6):573 - 80.

[2] Compagno, J., Oertel, J. E. Microcystic adenomas of the pancreas (glycogen-rich cystadenomas): a clinicopathologic study of 34 cases. *American journal of clinical pathology*, 1978; 69(3):289 - 98.

[3] Hodgkinson, D. J., ReMine, W. H., Weiland, L. H. A clinicopathologic study of 21 cases of pancreatic cystadenocarcinoma. *Annals of surgery*, 1978; 188(5):679 - 84.

[4] Kloppel, G., Kosmahl, M. Cystic lesions and neoplasms of the pancreas. The features are becoming clearer. *Pancreatology: official journal of the International Association of Pancreatology,* 2001; 1(6):648 - 55.

[5] Brugge, W. R., Lauwers, G. Y., Sahani, D., Fernandez-del Castillo, C., Warshaw, A. L. Cystic neoplasms of the pancreas. *The New England journal of medicine,* 2004; 351(12):1218 - 26.

[6] Basturk, O., Coban, I., Adsay, N. V. Pancreatic cysts: pathologic classification, differential diagnosis, and clinical implications. *Archives of pathology and laboratory medicine*, 2009; 133(3): 423 - 38.

[7] Kosmahl, M., Pauser, U., Peters, K., Sipos, B., Luttges, J., Kremer, B., et al. Cystic neoplasms of the pancreas and tumor-like lesions with cystic features: a review of 418 cases and a classification proposal. *Virchows Archiv: an international journal of pathology,* 2004; 445(2):168 - 78.

[8] de Jong, K., Bruno, M. J., Fockens, P. Epidemiology, diagnosis, and management of cystic lesions of the pancreas. *Gastroenterology research and practice,* 2012; 2012:147465.

[9] Farrell, J. J., Fernandez-del Castillo, C. Pancreatic cystic neoplasms: management and unanswered questions. *Gastroenterology,* 2013; 144(6):1303 - 15.

[10] Becker, W. F., Welsh, R. A., Pratt, H. S. Cystadenoma and Cystadenocarcinoma of the Pancreas. *Annals of surgery,* 1965; 161:845 - 63.

[11] Lim, S. J., Alasadi, R., Wayne, J. D., Rao, S., Rademaker, A., Bell, R., et al. Preoperative evaluation of pancreatic cystic lesions: cost-benefit analysis and proposed management algorithm. *Surgery,* 2005; 138(4):672 - 9; discussion 9 - 80.

[12] Fernandez-del Castillo, C., Targarona, J., Thayer, S. P., Rattner, D. W., Brugge, W. R., Warshaw, A. L. Incidental pancreatic cysts: clinicopathologic characteristics and comparison with symptomatic patients. *Archives of surgery*, 2003; 138(4):427 - 3; discussion 33 - 4.

[13] Laffan, T. A., Horton, K. M., Klein, A. P., Berlanstein, B., Siegelman, S. S., Kawamoto, S., et al. Prevalence of unsuspected pancreatic cysts on MDCT. *AJR American journal of roentgenology*, 2008; 191(3):802 - 7.

[14] Lee, H. J., Kim, M. J., Choi, J. Y., Hong, H. S., Kim, K. A. Relative accuracy of CT and MRI in the differentiation of benign from malignant pancreatic cystic lesions. *Clinical radiology,* 2011; 66(4): 315 - 21.

[15] Zhang, X. M., Mitchell, D. G., Dohke, M., Holland, G. A., Parker, L. Pancreatic cysts: depiction on single-shot fast spin-echo MR images. *Radiology,* 2002; 223(2):547 - 53.

[16] Spinelli, K. S., Fromwiller, T. E., Daniel, R. A., Kiely, J. M., Nakeeb, A., Komorowski, R. A., et al. Cystic pancreatic neoplasms: observe or operate. *Annals of surgery*, 2004; 239(5):651 - 7; discussion 7 - 9.

[17] de Jong, K., Nio, C. Y., Hermans, J. J., Dijkgraaf, M. G., Gouma, D. J., van Eijck, C. H., et al. High prevalence of pancreatic cysts detected by screening magnetic resonance imaging examinations. *Clinical gastroenterology and hepatology: the official clinical practice journal of the American Gastroenterological Association,* 2010; 8(9):806 - 11.

[18] Lee, K. S., Sekhar, A., Rofsky, N. M., Pedrosa, I. Prevalence of incidental pancreatic cysts in the adult population on MR imaging. *The American journal of gastroenterology*, 2010; 105(9):2079 - 84.
[19] Karoumpalis, I., Christodoulou, D. K. Cystic lesions of the pancreas. *Annals of gastroenterology: quarterly publication of the Hellenic Society of Gastroenterology*, 2016; 29(2):155 - 61.
[20] Sahani, D. V., Kambadakone, A., Macari, M., Takahashi, N., Chari, S., Fernandez-del Castillo, C. Diagnosis and management of cystic pancreatic lesions. *AJR American journal of roentgenology*, 2013; 200(2):343 - 54.
[21] Sahani, D. V., Miller, J. C., del Castillo, C. F., Brugge, W. R., Thrall, J. H., Lee, S. I. Cystic pancreatic lesions: classification and management. *Journal of the American College of Radiology: JACR,* 2009; 6(5):376 - 80.
[22] Kimura, W., Nagai, H., Kuroda, A., Muto, T., Esaki, Y. Analysis of small cystic lesions of the pancreas. *International journal of pancreatology: official journal of the International Association of Pancreatology,* 1995; 18(3):197 - 206.
[23] Valsangkar, N. P., Morales-Oyarvide, V., Thayer, S. P., Ferrone, C. R., Wargo, J. A., Warshaw, A. L., et al. 851 resected cystic tumors of the pancreas: a 33-year experience at the Massachusetts General Hospital. *Surgery*, 2012; 152(3 Suppl. 1):S4 - 12.
[24] Garud, S. S., Willingham, F. F. Molecular analysis of cyst fluid aspiration in the diagnosis and risk assessment of cystic lesions of the pancreas. *Clinical and translational science*, 2012; 5(1):102 - 7.
[25] Aaltonen, L. A. HSE. World Health Organization Classification of Tumours. Pathology and Genetics of Tumours of the Digestive System. *IARC Press*, Lyon, France. 2000.
[26] Zamboni, G. K. G., Hruban, R. H., et, al. Mucinous cystic neoplasms of the pancreas. In: World Health Organization Classification of Tumours. Pathology and Genetics of Tumours of the Digestive System. *IARC Press*, Lyon, France, 2000:p.234.
[27] Galanis, C., Zamani, A., Cameron, J. L., Campbell, K. A., Lillemoe, K. D., Caparrelli, D., et al. Resected serous cystic neoplasms of the

pancreas: a review of 158 patients with recommendations for treatment. *Journal of gastrointestinal surgery: official journal of the Society for Surgery of the Alimentary Tract*, 2007; 11(7):820 - 6.

[28] Tseng, J. F., Warshaw, A. L., Sahani, D. V., Lauwers, G. Y., Rattner, D. W., Fernandez-del Castillo, C. Serous cystadenoma of the pancreas: tumor growth rates and recommendations for treatment. *Annals of surgery*, 2005; 242(3):413 - 9; discussion 9 - 21.

[29] Le Borgne, J., de Calan, L., Partensky, C. Cystadenomas and cystadenocarcinomas of the pancreas: a multiinstitutional retrospective study of 398 cases. French Surgical Association. *Annals of surgery,* 1999; 230(2):152 - 61.

[30] Bassi, C., Salvia, R., Molinari, E., Biasutti, C., Falconi, M., Pederzoli, P. Management of 100 consecutive cases of pancreatic serous cystadenoma: wait for symptoms and see at imaging or vice versa? *World journal of surgery*, 2003; 27(3):319 - 23.

[31] Pyke, C. M., van Heerden, J. A., Colby, T. V., Sarr, M. G., Weaver, A. L. The spectrum of serous cystadenoma of the pancreas. Clinical, pathologic, and surgical aspects. *Annals of surgery*, 1992; 215(2):132 - 9. Epub 1992/02/01.

[32] Lundstedt, C., Dawiskiba, S. Serous and mucinous cystadenoma/ cystadenocarcinoma of the pancreas. *Abdominal imaging,* 2000; 25(2):201 - 6. Epub 2000/02/17.

[33] Matsumoto, T., Hirano, S., Yada, K., Shibata, K., Sasaki, A., Kamimura, T., et al. Malignant serous cystic neoplasm of the pancreas: report of a case and review of the literature. *Journal of clinical gastroenterology,* 2005; 39(3):253 - 6. Epub 2005/02/19.

[34] Federle, M. P., McGrath, K. M. Cystic neoplasms of the pancreas. *Gastroenterology clinics of North America*, 2007; 36(2):365 - 76, ix.

[35] Compton, C. C. Serous cystic tumors of the pancreas. *Seminars in diagnostic pathology*, 2000; 17(1):43 - 55.

[36] Crippa, S., Salvia, R., Warshaw, A. L., Dominguez, I., Bassi, C., Falconi, M., et al. Mucinous cystic neoplasm of the pancreas is not an aggressive entity: lessons from 163 resected patients. *Annals of surgery,* 2008; 247(4):571 - 9.

[37] Wilentz, R. E., Albores-Saavedra, J., Hruban, R. H. Mucinous cystic neoplasms of the pancreas. *Seminars in diagnostic pathology*, 2000; 17(1):31 - 42.

[38] Tanaka, M., Chari, S., Adsay, V., Fernandez-del Castillo, C., Falconi, M., Shimizu, M., et al. International consensus guidelines for management of intraductal papillary mucinous neoplasms and mucinous cystic neoplasms of the pancreas. *Pancreatology: official journal of the International Association of Pancreatology*, 2006; 6(1-2):17 - 32. Epub 2005/12/06.

[39] Zamboni, G., Scarpa, A., Bogina, G., Iacono, C., Bassi, C., Talamini, G., et al. Mucinous cystic tumors of the pancreas: clinicopathological features, prognosis, and relationship to other mucinous cystic tumors. *The American journal of surgical pathology*, 1999; 23(4):410 - 22.

[40] Adsay, N. V., Klimstra, D. S., Compton, C. C. Cystic lesions of the pancreas. Introduction. Seminars in diagnostic pathology, 2000; 17(1):1 - 6.

[41] Reddy, R. P., Smyrk, T. C., Zapiach, M., Levy, M. J., Pearson, R. K., Clain, J. E., et al. Pancreatic mucinous cystic neoplasm defined by ovarian stroma: demographics, clinical features, and prevalence of cancer. *Clinical gastroenterology and hepatology: the official clinical practice journal of the American Gastroenterological Association,* 2004; 2(11):1026 - 31.

[42] Del Chiaro, M., Verbeke, C., Salvia, R., Kloppel, G., Werner, J., McKay, C., et al. European experts consensus statement on cystic tumours of the pancreas. *Digestive and liver disease: official journal of the Italian Society of Gastroenterology and the Italian Association for the Study of the Liver,* 2013; 45(9):703 - 11.

[43] Crippa, S., Fernandez-Del Castillo, C., Salvia, R., Finkelstein, D., Bassi, C., Dominguez, I., et al. Mucin-producing neoplasms of the pancreas: an analysis of distinguishing clinical and epidemiologic characteristics. *Clinical gastroenterology and hepatology: the official clinical practice journal of the American Gastroenterological Association*, 2010; 8(2):213 - 9.

[44] Sohn, T. A., Yeo, C. J., Cameron, J. L., Hruban, R. H., Fukushima, N., Campbell, K. A., et al. Intraductal papillary mucinous neoplasms of the pancreas: an updated experience. *Annals of surgery,* 2004; 239(6):788 - 97; discussion 97 - 9.

[45] Kobari, M., Egawa, S., Shibuya, K., Shimamura, H., Sunamura, M., Takeda, K., et al. Intraductal papillary mucinous tumors of the pancreas comprise 2 clinical subtypes: differences in clinical characteristics and surgical management. *Archives of surgery,* 1999; 134(10):1131 - 6.

[46] Sugiyama, M., Izumisato, Y., Abe, N., Masaki, T., Mori, T., Atomi, Y. Predictive factors for malignancy in intraductal papillary-mucinous tumours of the pancreas. *The British journal of surgery,* 2003; 90(10):1244 - 9.

[47] Shimizu, Y., Yasui, K., Morimoto, T., Torii, A., Yamao, K., Ohhashi, K. Case of intraductal papillary mucinous tumor (noninvasive adenocarcinoma) of the pancreas resected 27 years after onset. *International journal of pancreatology: official journal of the International Association of Pancreatology*, 1999; 26(2):93 - 8.

[48] Adsay, N. V., Conlon, K. C., Zee, S. Y., Brennan, M. F., Klimstra, D. S. Intraductal papillary-mucinous neoplasms of the pancreas: an analysis of in situ and invasive carcinomas in 28 patients. *Cancer,* 2002; 94(1):62 - 77.

[49] Sugiyama, M., Atomi, Y. Extrapancreatic neoplasms occur with unusual frequency in patients with intraductal papillary mucinous tumors of the pancreas. *The American journal of gastroenterology,* 1999; 94(2):470 - 3.

[50] Sato, N., Rosty, C., Jansen, M., Fukushima, N., Ueki, T., Yeo, C. J., et al. STK11/LKB1 Peutz-Jeghers gene inactivation in intraductal papillary-mucinous neoplasms of the pancreas. *The American journal of pathology*, 2001; 159(6):2017 - 22.

[51] Maire, F., Hammel, P., Terris, B., Olschwang, S., O'Toole, D., Sauvanet, A., et al. Intraductal papillary and mucinous pancreatic tumour: a new extracolonic tumour in familial adenomatous polyposis. *Gut,* 2002; 51(3):446 - 9.

[52] Honselmann, K. C., Krauss, T., Geserick, S., Wellner, U. F., Wittel, U., Hopt, U. T., et al. Cystic lesions of the pancreas-is radical surgery really warranted? *Langenbeck's archives of surgery,* 2016; 401(4):449 - 56.

[53] Klimstra, D. S., Wenig, B. M., Heffess, C. S. Solid-pseudopapillary tumor of the pancreas: a typically cystic carcinoma of low malignant potential. *Seminars in diagnostic pathology*, 2000; 17(1):66 - 80. Epub 2000/03/18.

[54] Martin, R. C., Klimstra, D. S., Brennan, M. F., Conlon, K. C. Solid-pseudopapillary tumor of the pancreas: a surgical enigma? *Annals of surgical oncology,* 2002; 9(1):35 - 40. Epub 2002/02/09.

[55] Reddy, S., Cameron, J. L., Scudiere, J., Hruban, R. H., Fishman, E. K., Ahuja, N., et al. Surgical management of solid-pseudopapillary neoplasms of the pancreas (Franz or Hamoudi tumors): a large single-institutional series. *Journal of the American College of Surgeons*, 2009; 208(5):950 - 7; discussion 7 - 9.

[56] Butte, J. M., Brennan, M. F., Gonen, M., Tang, L. H., D'Angelica, M. I., Fong, Y., et al. Solid pseudopapillary tumors of the pancreas. Clinical features, surgical outcomes, and long-term survival in 45 consecutive patients from a single center. *Journal of gastrointestinal surgery: official journal of the Society for Surgery of the Alimentary Tract,* 2011; 15(2):350 - 7.

[57] Papavramidis, T., Papavramidis, S. Solid pseudopapillary tumors of the pancreas: review of 718 patients reported in English literature. *Journal of the American College of Surgeons*, 2005; 200(6):965 - 72. Epub 2005/06/01.

[58] Tipton, S. G., Smyrk, T. C., Sarr, M. G., Thompson, G. B. Malignant potential of solid pseudopapillary neoplasm of the pancreas. *The British journal of surgery,* 2006; 93(6):733 - 7. Epub 2006/04/13.

[59] Boninsegna, L., Partelli, S., D'Innocenzio, M. M., Capelli, P., Scarpa, A., Bassi, C., et al. Pancreatic cystic endocrine tumors: a different morphological entity associated with a less aggressive behavior. *Neuroendocrinology,* 2010; 92(4):246 - 51.

[60] Bordeianou, L., Vagefi, P. A., Sahani, D., Deshpande, V., Rakhlin, E., Warshaw, A. L., et al. Cystic pancreatic endocrine neoplasms: a distinct tumor type? *Journal of the American College of Surgeons,* 2008; 206(6):1154 - 8.

[61] Kloppel, G. Pseudocysts and other non-neoplastic cysts of the pancreas. Seminars in diagnostic pathology, 2000; 17(1):7 - 15.

[62] Zamboni, G., Terris, B., Scarpa, A., Kosmahl, M., Capelli, P., Klimstra, D. S., et al. Acinar cell cystadenoma of the pancreas: a new entity? *The American journal of surgical pathology*, 2002; 26(6):698-704.

[63] Albores-Saavedra, J. Acinar cystadenoma of the pancreas: a previously undescribed tumor. *Annals of diagnostic pathology,* 2002; 6(2):113 - 5.

Section II. Diagnostics

Section II. Diagnostics

In: Cystic Tumors of the Pancreas
Editor: Robert Grützmann
ISBN: 978-1-53612-523-8

Chapter 2

Clinical and Laboratory Diagnostic Parameters

Nikolaos Vassos**, MD, PhD, FACS
Department of Surgery, University Hospital Erlangen,
Erlangen, Germany

Abstract

Pancreatic cystic neoplasms (PCNs) represent a particularly interesting subset of pancreatic lesions showing a wide spectrum of clinical and histological features. Correct diagnosis and differentiation of these lesions is the pillar of clinical management because of the risk for concurrent or later development of malignancy. Clinical features are usually non-specific, whereas many patients are asymptomatic. Laboratory tests such as pancreatic enzymes and serum tumor markers are considered to be the most frequent and rapid method in diagnostics of PCNs. However, the determination of laboratory parameters is mostly used as a complementary method to other diagnostic techniques, since their role in predicting the malignant potential of PCNs remains controversial.

* Corresponding Author Email: Nikolaos.Vassos@uk-erlangen.de.

Keywords: pancreatic cystic neoplasms, symptoms, laboratory, serum, enzymes, tumor markers

INTRODUCTION

Pancreatic cystic neoplasms (PCNs) represent a particularly interesting subset of pancreatic lesions and are composed of a variety of neoplasms with a wide spectrum of histology and malignant potential. PCNs are categorized according to the World Health Organization histologic classification. Four main types of PCNs have been described: serous neoplasms, mucinous neoplasms, intraductal papillary cystic neoplasms and pseudopapillary cystic neoplasms [1-4].

These lesions present a diagnostic challenge to clinicians and laboratorians alike. A preoperative differential diagnosis of cystic lesions in the pancreas is very important given the presence of malignancy in some lesions at the time of presentation and the tendency to develop malignancy over time. Differentiation among serous cystadenomas (SCA), mucinous cystadenomas (MCA) or mucinous cystadenocarcinomas (MCAC), intraductal papillary cystic neoplasms (IPMN) and solid-pseudopapillary neoplasms (SPN) is crucial for the determination of the therapeutic strategy, but may be difficult because there are no reliable clinical and laboratory criteria to assist in making this differentiation. However, continuous improvement of the preoperative predictive abilities of cyst characteristics for determining malignancy has led to a more selective therapeutic approach [5-9].

CLINICAL PARAMETERS

Many patients with pancreatic cysts are asymptomatic (up to 40-75%) and the cystic mass is discovered only incidentally during diagnostic investigation of unrelated indications. When a patient is symptomatic, the presentation is usually non-specific and related to the mass effect of the neoplasm [10]. Symptomatic patients with PCN may present with jaundice, chronic abdominal pain, and recurrent pancreatitis (if obstruction is present), along with nonspecific symptoms of back pain, weight loss, anorexia, nausea and vomiting [10] (Table 1).

Table 1. Clinical features of patients with pancreatic cystic neoplasms

	Serous cystic tumor	Mucinous neoplasm	Main-duct intraductal papillary mucinous neoplasm	Branch-duct intraductal papillary mucinous neoplasm	Solid pseudopapillary neoplasm
Typical clinical presentation	Incidental or abdominal pain or mass effect	Incidental or abdominal pain or malignancy related	Incidental or pancreatitis or pancreatic insuffiency or malignancy related	Incidental or pancreatitis or malignancy related	Incidental or abdominal pain or mass effect

The symptoms of each type of PCN in detail are as follow:

Serous Cystic Tumor (SCN)

SCNs are usually asymptomatic and thus incidentally discovered [11]. As for symptoms, they are mostly not specific and often attributed to mass effects because of cyst enlargement and subsequent space occupation or to infiltration of adjacent structures [12-14]. Several studies have shown that cysts greater than 4 cm in size are more likely to cause symptoms or findings on physical examination if compared to pancreatic cysts <4 cm (72% *vs* 22%, $P<0.001$) [11, 15-18].

The most frequently reported clinical manifestations are abdominal discomfort and low-grade pain (47-75%). Weight loss, palpable mass, jaundice and obstruction of the upper gastrointestinal tract are less frequent or rare and are related to the location (e.g., jaundice) and the extensive growth of the lesion (e.g., palpable mass or obstruction of the upper GI) [1,

10, 14, 19, 20]. A history of acute or chronic pancreatitis is absent except in the rare patient in whom SCN causes an episode of acute pancreatitis, presumably due to partial pancreatic duct obstruction [2, 20]. A multinational study of the European Study Group on Cystic Tumors of the Pancreas including 2,622 cases of SCN revealed that patients could present with nonspecific abdominal pain (27%), pancreatic-biliary symptoms (9%), diabetes mellitus (5%), or other symptoms (4%), with the remaining patients being asymptomatic (61%) [21].

Mucinous Cystic Neoplasm (MCN)

The clinical presentations of MCNs can be extremely various. Almost half of the patients are asymptomatic and diagnosis is made incidentally. Symptoms in MCNs are non-specific. It has been reported that, even among asymptomatic patients, 18% already have early or invasive cancer, 42% have a potentially malignant lesion and 40% a benign lesion [22]. MCNs can present with abdominal pain, recurrent pancreatitis, gastric outlet obstruction, postprandial fullness and/or a palpable mass [16, 23]. Jaundice, weight loss and anorexia are considered to be worrisome symptoms, correlating with a higher likelihood of malignancy of the lesion [23, 24]. Generally, the duration of symptoms ranges from a few days of abdominal discomfort and pain to a 5-year history of an abdominal mass [25]. However, the presence of symptoms in patients with MCN increases the likelihood of a malignant MCN, but the absence of symptoms does not necessarily exclude it [20, 26].

Intraductal Papillary Mucinous Neoplasm (IPMN)

Clinically, three different varieties of IPMN exist: main duct type (MD-IPMN), characterized by diffuse dilatation of the main pancreatic duct, branch duct type (BD-IPMN) appearing as saccular or cystic dilatation of branch cysts, and mixed-type involving both [27]. As with the other pancreatic cystic lesions, many patients with IPMNs have no symptoms, with the neoplasm being detected incidentally when imaging studies are performed for unrelated indications [28, 29]. Common symptoms of IPMN at presentation include abdominal discomfort or pain (70-80%), nausea and vomiting (11-21%), back pain (10%), weight loss (20-40%), diabetes, jaundice, and acute pancreatitis. These symptoms are more frequently seen with MD-IPMN/mixed IPMN than BD-IPMN [29-33].

Approximately 20% of patients with IPMN present with acute pancreatitis of mild to moderate severity or with pancreatitis-like symptoms or even with symptoms suggestive of chronic pancreatitis (exocrine and endocrine pancreatic insufficiency, maldigestion), resulting from intermittent obstruction of the pancreatic duct with mucus plugs [30, 31, 34]. This is why IPMN can be mistaken for idiopathic pancreatitis when patients have a large, dilated pancreatic duct. However, patients with IPMN are typically older compared to patients with chronic pancreatitis and have no history of prolonged pancreatopathy [10].

When an invasive carcinoma coexists in IPMN (up to 40% of patients), a symptom profile similar to that of pancreatic ductal adenocarcinoma (pain, jaundice, weight loss, and malaise) may be present [10]. Symptomatic presentation of main duct disease generally collates with malignancy, since back pain, jaundice, weight loss, anorexia, steatorrhea and new onset diabetes are harbingers of malignancy and independent predictors for the presence of carcinoma [31, 35].

Solid-Pseudopapillary Neoplasm (SPN)

Due to its slow growth, SPN often remains asymptomatic, until the tumor has enlarged considerably [36, 37]. In the past, approximately 80% of patients with SPN were symptomatic. However, incidental detection of SPNs during imaging for unrelated diseases or after a blunt abdominal trauma is becoming more common with the increased use of radiologic assessments and accounts for up to 50% of cases [37-41].

The clinical presentation of SPNs is not specific. Most of patients present with non-specific symptoms including abdominal discomfort, mild abdominal pain, palpable abdominal mass (most common presentation in children), followed by nausea, vomiting and weight loss [41, 42]. Other symptoms that occur less frequently include gastrointestinal obstruction, anemia, jaundice, and pancreatitis or very rarely jaundice and hematemesis [40, 42].

Laboratory Parameters

Laboratory tests such as the assessment of pancreatic enzymes and tumor markers are considered to be a frequent, economic, convenient and rapid method in the diagnostics of PCNs.

Pancreatic Enzymes

Although in some patients there may be elevations of pancreatic enzymes (amylase, lipase) with episodes of pain (with or without biliary obstruction), in most cases routine laboratory tests are normal. Sperti et al., showed that amylase and lipase levels in serum were not statistically different in four groups of patients with PCNs [43]. Sensitivity of serum enzymes in detecting pancreatic pseudocysts was extremely low (amylase: 48% and lipase: 38%), whereas specificity was 85% and 81%, and positive predictive value (PPV) 71% and 61% respectively [43].

Serum pancreatic enzymes outside the normal range (greater than normal) are associated with a greater risk of malignancy and invasiveness in patients with IPMN, especially in patients without a history of acute pancreatitis ($p = .003$) [44]. This is why several authors suggest that serum pancreatic enzymes level may be a more accurate predictor of malignancy/invasiveness (risk of invasive disease) than pancreatitis [45, 46].

Serum Tumor Markers

Serum tumor markers have been routinely used in the preoperative workup of patients with pancreatic cancer since they are elevated in late-stage pancreatic malignancy. But they often fail to discern between benign and pre-malignant cysts because they may remain within reference values regardless of the nature of the lesion. This is why the utility of serum tumor markers in PCNs is limited [47]. A specific serum tumor marker, able to discriminate the different types of PCNs, is not yet available. Early studies in the 1980s supposed the role of carcinoembryonic antigen (CEA) and carbohydrate antigen (CA) 19-9 in the differentiation of PCNs [31, 48]. During the last years, the role of serum tumor markers in differentiating cyst types and predicting malignancy has been intensively researched and several follow-up reports and multiple studies have downplayed their utility and supported the use of serum CEA and CA 19-9 [43, 48-51].

Looking at CEA status alone, Bassi et al., reported that serum CEA levels are elevated in mucinous cystic neoplasms (MCNs), compared to serous cystic neoplasms (SCNs) [47]. This finding had a high specificity and but a low sensitivity; however positive predictive value (PPV) revealed that, when positive, CEA level could help to distinguish MCNs from other PCNs and may predict malignancy without any statistical significance [47]. Hoffman et al., also reported that the proportion of elevated serum CEA (normal serum CEA $<$5ng/ml) measured in malignant and benign PCNs was not found to be significantly different ($p = 0.43$) [52].

Furthermore, Sperti et al., demonstrated that mean CEA levels were in the normal range for all types of PCNs. Nevertheless, SCN showed significantly lower CEA levels ($P < 0.02$) compared with the other types [43].

The role of serum CA 19-9 in distinguishing benign from malignant disease remains controversial but it could potentially be an initiatory and essential preoperative assessment in routine clinical practice. Several authors reported that elevated serum CA 19-9 is a significant high risk factor of malignant PCNs [43, 53-56]. Specifically, Hoffman et al., reported that median serum CA 19-9 measurements in the malignant and benign groups of PCNs were 20.5 ng/mL and 11.0 ng/mL, respectively (normal serum CA 19-9 <37.0 ng/mL) without any statistical significance. Besides, the proportion of elevated serum tumor markers measured in malignant and benign neoplasms was also not significantly different (p = 0.26) [52]. However, Sperti et al., demonstrated that mean CA 19-9 levels were significantly elevated in the patients with MCNs compared with other PCNs (sensitivity and specificity of serum CA 19-9 in detecting MCNs: 75% and 96% respectively) [43]. Furthermore, in a recent meta-analysis, Cao et al., indicated that serum CA 19-9 could be a useful tool with high pooled specificity for discriminating benign from malignant PCN and predicting their behavior [57]. However a significant number of malignant PCNs might be misdiagnosed as benign disease when only relying on serum CA 19-9.

Interstingly, serum CA 19-9 is elevated in less than 20% of cases of noninvasive IPMN and, if elevated, are suggestive of malignant transformation [53, 58-61]. Serum CA 19-9 is also a useful non-invasive tool for distinguishing malignant IPMNs, and should be taken into account in the decision for or against surgery, although other studies revealed that neither serum CA 19-9 nor CEA were able to provide evidence for or against resection [52]. Concerning diagnostics of SPN, serum tumor markers are of no help [37, 40].

A multivariate analysis identified elevation of serum CEA or Ca 19-9 as independent predictors of a malignant PCN (p = 0.014, sensitivity 43% and specificity 88%) [62]. Interestingly, elevation of serum CEA and Ca 19-9 was more accurate than elevation of either tumor marker alone. Goh et al., showed in this analysis that mean value of elevated serum CEA was 5.5 ng/ml in MCNs, 2.6 ng/ml in SCNs, 5.0 ng/ml in IPMNs and 2.0 ng/ml in SPNs; whereas the mean value of elevated serum CA 19-9 was 396 ng/ml in MCNs, 215 ng/ml in SCNs, 60 ng/ml in IPMNs and 16 ng/ml in SPNs, suggesting a potential predictive value of this serum tumor marker (high PPV and specificity but poor sensitivity) [62].

Other serum tumor markers (Ca 15-3, Ca 125 and Ca 72-4) were also studied by several authors but they were always negative in all types of

PCNs and particularly in both tumor groups (mucinous and nonmucinous neoplasms) [47, 50].

Regarding the differentiation between SCNs and MCNs, Bassi et al., analyzed a combination of measurements of serum tumor markers (CEA, CA 19-9, Ca 125) since no single serum tumor marker could differentiate MCN from SCN [52]. Using the presence of two or more abnormal serum CEA, Ca 19-9, or Ca 125 levels as an indication of MCN, the sensitivity in differentiating MCN from SCN was increased to 27% and the specificity and PPV were 100%, but without statistical significance [47]. It was suggested that a positive CEA serum marker status and/or positivity of more than two markers (CEA, Ca 19-9, and/or Ca 19-9) have a good specificity for differentiating MCNs from other PCNs and could predict the presence of a malignant tumor [44, 47, 63]. The real value of these tests lies in their ability to detect MCNs because all three markers being positive occurred exclusively in MCACs, and this could be used to differentiate MCAs from MCACs [47]. Bassi et al., proposed that all cystic lesions which do not involve the pancreatic duct and have no clinical signs of an endocrine syndrome and have a positive CEA level or more than two positive serum markers (CEA, Ca 19-9, and/or Ca 125), should be considered MCNs [47].

CONCLUSION

A preoperative differential diagnosis of cystic lesions of the pancreas is very important for the determination of the therapeutic strategy. Differentiation among PCNs is difficult on the basis of a clinical presentation. Laboratory tests (pancreatic enzymes and serum tumor markers) deserve to be widely used as complementary to other diagnostic techniques, since they have been reported as useful parameters and are considered as an economic, convenient, safe and rapid method in diagnostics of PCNs. However, the role of serum tumor marker expression in distinguishing between benign and malignant diseases remains controversial, and more sensitive biomarkers are needed.

REFERENCES

[1] Salvia, R., Festa, L., Butturini, F., et al. Pancreatic cystic tumors. *Minerva Chir.* 2004;59:185-207.

[2] Becker Welsh, R. A., Pratt, H. S. Cystadenoma and cystadenocarcinoma of pancreas. *Ann. Surg.* 1965;161:845-863.

[3] World Health Organization Classification of Tumours. Pathology and Genetics of Tumours of the Digestive System, Aaltonen, L. A., Hamilton, S. R. (Eds), *IARC Press*, Lyon, France 2000.

[4] Zamboni, G., Kloeppel, G., Hruban, R. H., et al. Mucinous cystic neoplasms of the pancreas. In: World Health Organization Classification of Tumours. Pathology and Genetics of Tumours of the Digestive System, Aaltonen LA, Hamilton SR (Eds), *IARC Press*, Lyon, France 2000. p.234.

[5] Allen, P. J., D'Angelica, M., Gonen, M., et al. A selective approach to the resection of cystic lesions of the pancreas: results from 539 consecutive patients. *Ann. Surg.* 2006;244:572-582.

[6] Horvath, K. D., Chabot, J. A.. An aggressive resectional approach to cystic neoplasms of the pancreas. *Am. J. Surg.* 1999;178:269-274.

[7] Allen, P. J., Jaques, D. P., D'Angelica, M., et al. Cystic lesions of the pancreas: selection criteria for operative and nonoperative management in 209 patients. *J. Gastrointest. Surg.* 2003;7:970-977.

[8] Grobmyer, S. R., Cance, W. G., Copeland, E. M., et al. Hochwald Is there an indication for initial conservative management of pancreatic cystic lesions? *J. Surg. Oncol.* 2009;100:372-374.

[9] Khalid, A., Brugge, W. ACG practice guidelines for the diagnosis and management of neoplastic pancreatic cysts. *Am. J. Gastroenterol.* 2007;102:2339-2349.

[10] Sakorafas, G. H., Sarr, M. G. Cystic neoplasms of the pancreas; what a clinician should know. *Cancer Treat. Rev.* 2005;31:507-535.

[11] Tseng, J. F., Warshaw, A. L., Sahani, D. V., et al. Serous cystadenoma of the pancreas: tumor growth rates and recommendations for treatment. *Ann. Surg.* 2005;242:413-419.

[12] Pyke, C. M., van Heerden, J. A., Colby, T. V., et al. The spectrum of serous cystadenoma of the pancreas. Clinical, pathologic, and surgical aspects. *Ann. Surg.* 1992;215:132.

[13] Lundste, C, Dawiskiba, S. Serous and mucinous cystadenoma/cyst adenocarcinoma of the pancreas. *Abdom. Imaging*. 2000;25:201.

[14] Spinelli, K. S., Fromwiller, T. E., Daniel, R. A., et al. Cystic pancreatic neoplasms: observe or operate. *Ann. Surg.* 2004;239:651-657.

[15] Tseng, J. F., Warshaw, A. L., Sahani, D. V., et al. Serous cystadenoma of the pancreas: tumor growth rates and recommendations for treatment. *Ann. Surg.* 2005;242:413.

[16] Sharma, A. Tumors of the Pancreas. In: *Current Diagnosis & Treatment: Gastroenterology, Hepatology, & Endoscopy*, Greenberger, N. J., Blumberg, R. S., Burakoff, R. (Eds), McGraw-Hill, New York 2009. p.318.

[17] El-Hayek, K. M., Brown, N., O'Rourke, C., et al. Rate of growth of pancreatic serous cystadenoma as an indication for resection. *Surgery* 2013;154:794-800.

[18] Fukasawa, M., Maguchi, H., Takahashi, K., et al. Clinical features and natural history of serous cystic neoplasm of the pancreas. *Pancreatology* 2010;10:695-701.

[19] Pyke, C. M., van Heerden, J. A., Colby, T. V., et al. The spectrum of serous cystadenoma of the pancreas. Clinical, pathologic and surgical aspects. *Ann. Surg.* 1992;215:132-139.

[20] Jeurnink, S. M., Vleggaar, F. P., Siersema, P. D. Overview of the clinical problem: Facts and current issues of mucinous cystic neoplasms of the pancreas. *Dig. Liver Dis*. 2008;40:837-846.

[21] Jais, B., Rebours, V., Malleo, G., et al. Serous cystic neoplasm of the pancreas: a multinational study of 2622 patients under the auspices of the International Association of Pancreatology and European Pancreatic Club (European Study Group on Cystic Tumors of the Pancreas) *Gut* 2016;65:305-312.

[22] Fernadez-del, C. C., Targarona, J., Thayer, S. P., et al. Incidental pancreatic cysts: clinicopathologic characteristics and comparison with symptomatic patients. *Arch. Surg.* 2003;138:427-433.

[23] Valsangkar, N. P., Morales-Oyarvide, V., Thayer, S. P., et al. 851 resected cystic tumors of the pancreas: A 33-year experience at the Massachusetts General Hospital. *Surgery* 2012;152:4-12.

[24] Turner, B. G., Brugge, W. R. Pancreatic cystic lesions: when to watch, when to operate, and when to ignore. *Curr. Gastroenterol. Rep.* 2010;12:98-105.

[25] Compagno, J., Oertel, J. E. Microcystic adenomas of the pancreas (glycogen-rich cystadenomas): a clinicopatholoigc study of 34 cases. *Am. J. Clin. Pathol.* 1978;69:289-298.

[26] Sarr, M. G., Carpenter, H. A., Prabhakar, L. P., et al. Clinical and pathologic correlation of 84 mucinous cystic neoplasms of the pancreas: can one reliably differentiate benign from malignant (or premalignant) neoplasms? *Ann. Surg.* 2000;231:205-212.

[27] Hruban, R. H., Takaori, K., Klimstra, D. S., et al. An illustrated consencus on the classification of pancreatic intraepithelial neoplasia and intraductal papillary musinous neoplasms. *Am. J. Surg. Pathol.* 2004;28:977-987.

[28] Grützmann, R., Niedergethmann, M., Pilarsky, C., et al. Intraductal papillary mucinous tumors of the pancreas: biology, diagnosis, and treatment. *Oncologist* 2010; 15:1294.

[29] Sakorafas, G. H., Smyrniotis, V., Reid-Lombardo, K. M., et al. Primary pancreatic cystic neoplasms revisited. Part III. Intraductal papillary mucinous neoplasms. *Surg. Oncol.* 2011;20:109-118.

[30] Jang, J. W., Kim, M. H., Jeong, S. U., et al. Clinical characteristics of intraductal papillary mucinous neoplasm manifesting as acute pancreatitis or acute recurrent pancreatitis. *J. Gastroenterol. Hepatol.* 2013;28:731-738.

[31] Salvia, R., Fernandez-del Castillo, C., Bassi, C., et al. Main-duct intraductal papillary mucinous neoplasms of the pancreas: clinical predictors of malignancy and long-term survival following resection. *Ann. Surg.* 2004;239:678-685.

[32] Gourgiotis, S., Ridolfini, M. P., Germanos, S. Intraductal papillary mucinous neoplasms of the pancreas. *Eur. J. Surg. Oncol.* 2007;33:678-684.

[33] Tanaka, M., Kobayashi, K., Mizumoto, K. Clinical aspects of intraductal papillary mucinous neoplasm of the pancreas. *J. Gastroenterol.* 2005;40:669-675.

[34] Bassi, C., Procacci, C., Zamboni, G., et al. Intraductal papillary mucinous tumors of the pancreas. Verona University Pancreatic Team. *Int. J. Pancreatol.* 2000; 27:181.

[35] D'Angelica, M., Brennan, M. F., Suriawinata, A. A., et al. Intraductal papillary mucinous neoplasms of the pancreas: an analysis of clinicopathologic features and outcome. *Ann. Surg.* 2004;239:400-408.

[36] Chen, X., Zhou, G. W., Zhou, H. J., et al. Diagnosis and treatment of solid-pseudopapillary tumors of the pancreas. *Hepatobiliary Pancreat. Dis. Int.* 2005;4:456-459.

[37] Vassos, N., Agaimy, A., Klein, P., et al. Solid-pseudopapillary neoplasm (SPN) of the pancreas: case series and literature review on an enigmatic entity. *Int. J. Clin. Exp. Pathol.* 2013;6:1051-1059.

[38] Mozaffar, M., Abdollahi, S. M. Acute post-traumatic presentation of a solid-pseudopapillary tumor of the pancreas: a case report. *Iran. J. Cancer Prev.* 2008;1:43-51.

[39] Igbinosa, O. Pseudopapillary tumor of the pancreas. An algorithmic approach. *JOP* 2011;12:262-265.

[40] Papavramidis, T., Papavramidis, S. Solid pseudopapillary tumors of the pancreas: Review of 718 patients reported in English literature. *J. Am. Coll. Surg. 2005*;200:965-972.

[41] Romics, L. Jr., Oláh, A., Belágyi, T., et al. Solid pseudopapillary neoplasm of the pancreas-proposed algorithms for diagnosis and surgical treatment. *Langenbecks Arch. Surg*. 2010; 395:747.

[42] Reddy, S., Cameron, J. L., Scudiere, J., et al. Surgical management of solid-pseudopapillary neoplasms of the pancreas: a large single-institutional series. *J. Amer. Coll. Surg.* 2009;208:950-959.

[43] Sperti, C., Pasquali, C., Guolo, P., et al. Serum tumor markers and cyst fluid analysis are useful for the diagnosis of pancreatic cystic tumors. *Cancer* 1996;78:237-243.

[44] Roch, A., Parikh, A., Al-Haddad, M. A., et al. Abnormal serum pancreatic enzymes, but not pancreatitis, are associated with an increased risk of malignancy in patients with intraductal papillary mucinous neoplasms. *Surgery* 2014;156:923-929.

[45] Tanaka, M., Chari, S., Adsay, V., et al. International consensus guidelines for management of intraductal papillary mucinous neoplasms and mucinous cystic neoplasms of the pancreas. *Pancreatology* 2006;6:17-32

[46] Tanaka, M., Fernandez del Castillo, C., Adsay, V., et al. International consensus guidelines 2012 for management of IPMN and MCN of pancreas. *Pancreatology* 2012;12:183-197.

[47] Bassi, C., Salvia, R., Gumbs, A. A., et al. The value of standard serum tumor markers in differentiating mucinous from serous cystic tumors of the pancreas: CEA, Ca 19-9, Ca 125, Ca 15-3. *Langenbecks Arch. Surg.* 2002;387:281-285.

[48] Tansuta, M., Iishi, H., Ichii, M., et al. Values of carcinoembryonic antigen, elastase 1 and carbohydrate antigen determinant in aspirated pancreatic cystic fluid in the diagnosis of cysts of the pancreas. *Cancer* 1986;57:1836-1839.

[49] Sugiyama, M., Izumisato, Y., Abe, N., et al. Predictive factors for malignancy in intraductal papillary-mucinous tumors of the pancreas. *Br. J. Surg.* 2003;90:1244-1249.

[50] Goh, B. K., Tan, D. M., Thng, C. H., et al. Are the Sendai and Fukuoka Consensus Guidelines for cystic mucinous neoplasms of the pancreas useful in the initial triage of all suspected pancreatic cystic neoplasms? A single-institution experience with 317 surgically-treated patients. *Ann. Surg. Oncol.* 2014;21:1919-1926.

[51] Javle, M., Shah, P., Yu, J., et al. Cystic pancreatic tumors (CPT): predictors of malignant behavior. *J. Surg. Oncol.* 2007;95:221-228.

[52] Hoffman, R. L., Gates, J. L., Kochman, M. L., et al. Analysis of cyst size and tumor markers in the management of pancreatic cysts:

support for the original Sendai criteria. *J. Am. Coll. Surg.* 2015;220:1087-1095.

[53] Fritz, S., Hackert, T., Hinz, U., et al. Role of serum carbohydrate antigen 19–9 and carcinoembryonic antigen in distinguishing between benign and invasive intraductal papillary mucinous neoplasm of the pancreas. *Br. J. Surg.* 2011;98(1):104-110.

[54] Hwang, D. W., Jang, J., Lim, C., et al. Determination of Malignant and Invasive Predictors in Branch Duct Type Intraductal Papillary Mucinous Neoplasms of the Pancreas: A Suggested Scoring Formula. *J. Korean Med. Sci.* 2011;26:740.

[55] Pasquali, C., Sperti, C., Alfano, D'Andrea A., et al. Evaluation of carbohydrate antigens 19-9 and 12-5 in patients with pancreatic cancer. *Paticreas* 1987;2:234-237.

[56] Steinberg, W. The clinical utility of the CA 19-9 tumor associated antigen. *An. J. Gastroenterol.* 1990;85:350-355.

[57] Cao, S., Hu, Y., Gao, X., et al. Serum carbohydrate antigen 19-9 in differential diagnosis of benign and malignant pancreatic cystic neoplasms: a meta-analysis. *PLoS One* 2016;11:e0166406.

[58] Fritz, S., Hackert, T., Hinz, U., et al. Role of serum carbohydrate antigen 19-9 and carcinoembryonic antigen in distinguishing between benign and invasive intraductal papillary mucinous neoplasm of the pancreas. *Br. J. Surg*. 2011;98:104.

[59] Schmidt, C. M., White, P. B., Waters, J. A., et al. Intraductal papillary mucinous neoplasms: predictors of malignant and invasive pathology. *Ann. Surg.* 2007;246:644-654.

[60] Grobmyer, S. R., Cance, W. G., Copeland, E. M., et al. Is there an indication for initial conservative management of pancreatic cystic lesions? *J. Surg. Oncol.* 2009;100:372-374.

[61] Sultana, A., Jackson, R., Tim, G., et al. What Is the Best Way to Identify Malignant Transformation Within Pancreatic IPMN: A Systematic Review and Meta-Analyses. *Clin. Transl. Gastroenterol.* 2015;6(e130).

[62] Goh, B. K., Tan, Y. M., Thng, C. H., et al. How useful are clinical, biochemical and cross-sectional imaging features in predicting

potentially malignant or malignant cystic lesions of the pancreas. Results from a single institution experience with 220 surgically treated patients. *J. Am. Coll. Surg.* 2008;206:17-27.

[63] Le Borgne, J., de Calan, L., Partensky, C. French Surgical Association. Cystadenomas and cystadenocarcinomas of the pancreas. A multi-institutional retrospective study of 398 cases. *Ann. Surg*. 1999;230:152-161.

In: Cystic Tumors of the Pancreas
Editor: Robert Grützmann
ISBN: 978-1-53612-523-8

Chapter 3

IMAGING OF CYSTIC PANCREATIC TUMORS

Verena Plodeck, MD*
Department of Radiology, University Hospital Dresden, Germany

ABSTRACT

Cystic lesions of the pancreas constitute a common (incidental) finding on imaging. Since there is a variety of cystic tumors requiring different therapeutic approaches, accurate diagnosis is vital prior to treatment planning. An in-depth knowledge of the most common cystic entities as well as their typical imaging criteria is necessary to establish the correct diagnosis and subsequently initiate appropriate treatment.

Keywords: cystic pancreatic lesions, imaging, ultrasound, CT, MRI, MRCP

* Corresponding Author Email: Verena.Plodeck@uniklinikum-dresden.de.

INTRODUCTION

Cystic lesions of the pancreas are common findings and frequently detected incidentally during an abdominal ultrasound, CT or MRI imaging [1, 2, 3]. Since cystic pancreatic lesions range from benign (e.g., pseudocysts) to malignant (e.g., cystic neuroendocrine tumors), imaging plays an important role in the diagnosis of cystic lesions and subsequent treatment planning. Patient history and clinical as well as laboratory parameters are vital in the differential diagnosis of pancreatic lesions and should therefore always be readily available to the radiologist.

If cystic pancreatic lesions are detected on imaging, the position of the lesion should be noted, since some entities are more common in certain parts of the pancreas; for example, mucinous cystic neoplasms are more commonly seen in the pancreatic tail [4]. As mentioned above, in finding a diagnosis patient data like gender is also relevant, as some lesions show a gender preference, e.g., solid pseudopapillary neoplasms are far more common in younger women than men [5]. Other imaging findings like signs of chronic pancreatitis, dilatation of the main pancreatic duct or multiple other cystic lesions of the pancreas are also important factors in establishing a diagnosis.

The following chapter will give an overview of the most commonly used imaging methods including ultrasound, CT, MRI and PET/CT/PET/MRI, whereas endosonography will be covered in the next chapter.

Patient history and clinical as well as laboratory parameters are vital in the differential diagnosis of pancreatic lesions. For example, pseudocysts should not be diagnosed without a prior history of pancreatitis.

ULTRASOUND

Ultrasound is the most commonly used imaging modality in abdominal imaging. Its advantages consist of the wide availability, easy handling and low costs, the disadvantages are limitations due to patient conditions (obesity, intestinal gas), the dependence on the examiner's experience as well as the reproducibility of the scan. In terms of planning a surgical procedure this might pose a challenge if the ultrasound was not performed by the operating surgeon himself. Contrast-enhanced [6] ultrasound can facilitate the differential diagnosis of cystic lesions and improve the detection of features suspicious for malignancy. Sensitivity and specificity of ultrasound varies greatly with patient characteristics as well as examiner's experience.

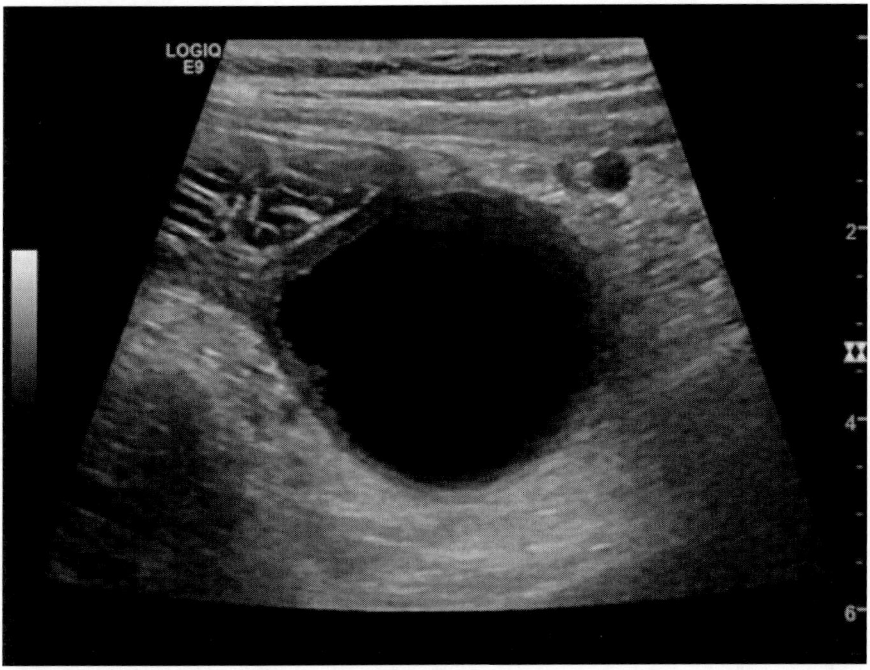

Figure 1. Ultrasound image demonstrating a cystic lesion with an irregular, thickened wall – Pancreatic pseudocyst (Image courtesy Sven Pannach, MD, Department of Medicine I, University Hospital Dresden).

CT

CT is also widely available and used for a multitude of indications. Cystic pancreatic lesions are a common (incidental) finding on CT and should be carefully assessed. The benefits of CT imaging are the short scanning time, the reproducibility of the imaging and low risk of artifacts, which renders it a good modality for surgical planning. The disadvantages include the higher costs compared to ultrasound, as well as radiation exposure. For the differential diagnosis of cystic lesions of the pancreas non-contrast enhanced CT scans are less useful than contrast-enhanced CT scans. The use of oral contrast (e.g., water or iodine-based/bariumsulfate compounds) and specific patient positioning (e.g., partial right lateral position) can be helpful [7]. The accuracy of CT for the characterization of cystic pancreatic lesions ranges from 56% to 85%, according to the literature [8, 9, 10, 11, 12].

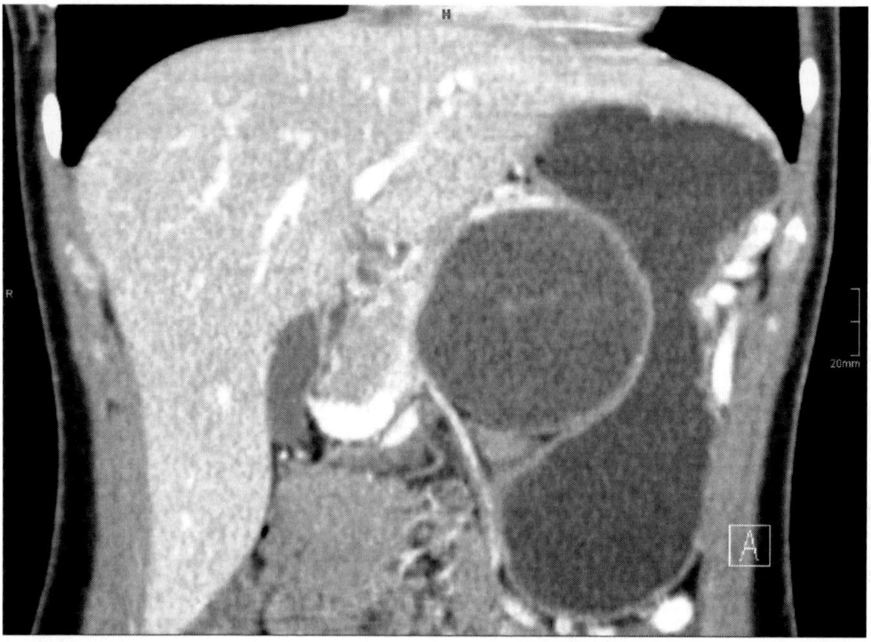

Figure 2. Coronal CT image of a large cystic lesion of the pancreatic tail, demonstrating septae - Mucinous cystic neoplasm.

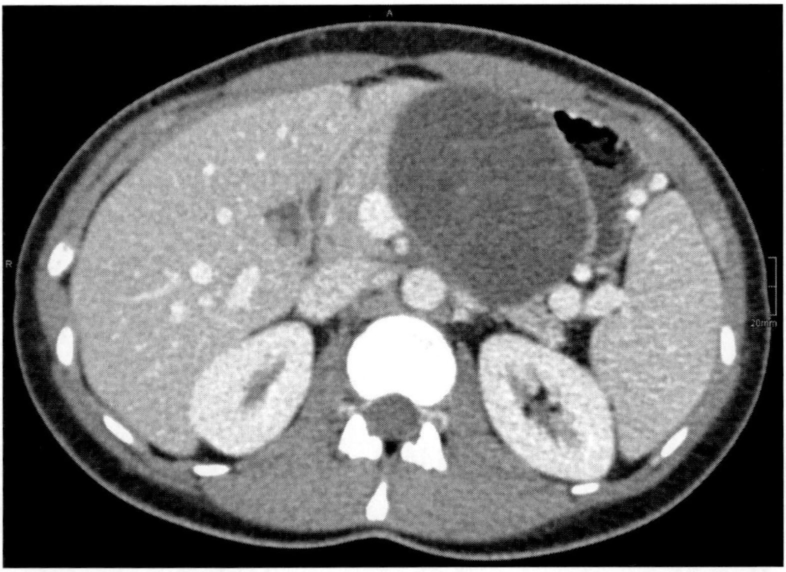

Figure 3. Axial CT image of a large cystic lesion of the pancreatic tail, demonstrating septae - Mucinous cystic neoplasm.

MRI

MRI is an imaging modality with excellent soft tissue contrast and therefore very useful in the differential diagnosis of cystic pancreatic lesions. Moreover, MRCP (magnetic resonance cholangiopancreatography) allows non-interventional imaging of the pancreatic duct system and demonstrates possible communication of lesions with the duct system. The good reproducibility and the above mentioned characteristics comprise the benefits of MRI imaging. The disadvantages are higher costs, reduced availability and MRI's propensity for artifacts. Contraindications like ferromagnetic implants or claustrophobia exclude some patients from MRI diagnostics. The combination of multiple MRI sequences (T1, T2 with and without fat saturation, diffusion-weighted imaging, contrast-enhanced sequences, MRCP etc.) allows for a thorough assessment of pancreatic lesions and facilitates the differential diagnosis. The accuracy of MRI in determining malignancy of a cystic pancreatic lesion varies between 73% to 91% [13, 14].

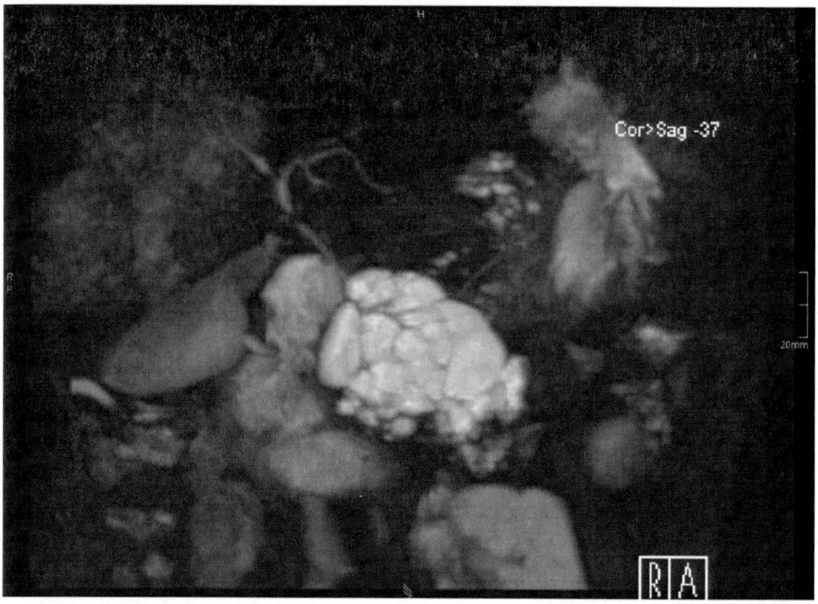

Figure 4. MRCP demonstrating a large multicystic lesion of the pancreatic head – Serous microcystic adenoma.

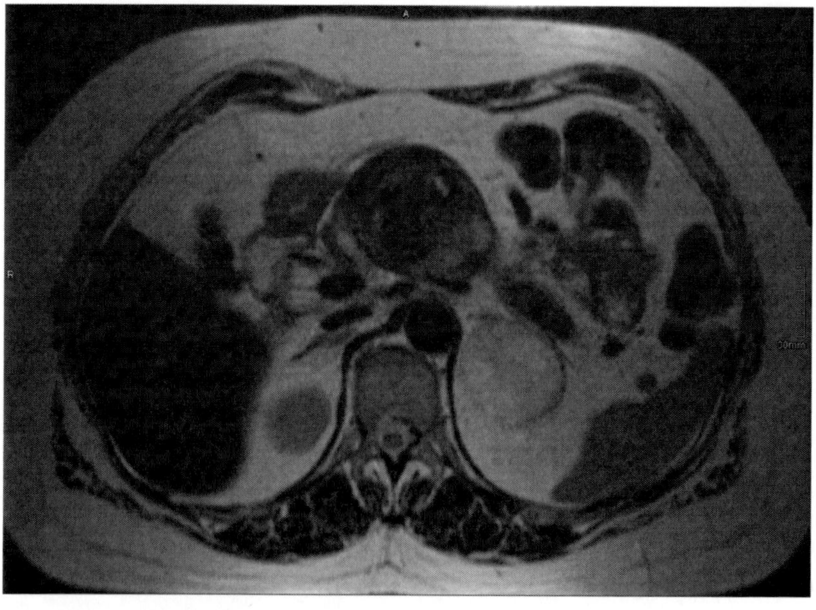

Figure 5. T2 weighted MRI image showing an inhomogenous lesion of the pancreatic body – Solid pseudopapillary neoplasm.

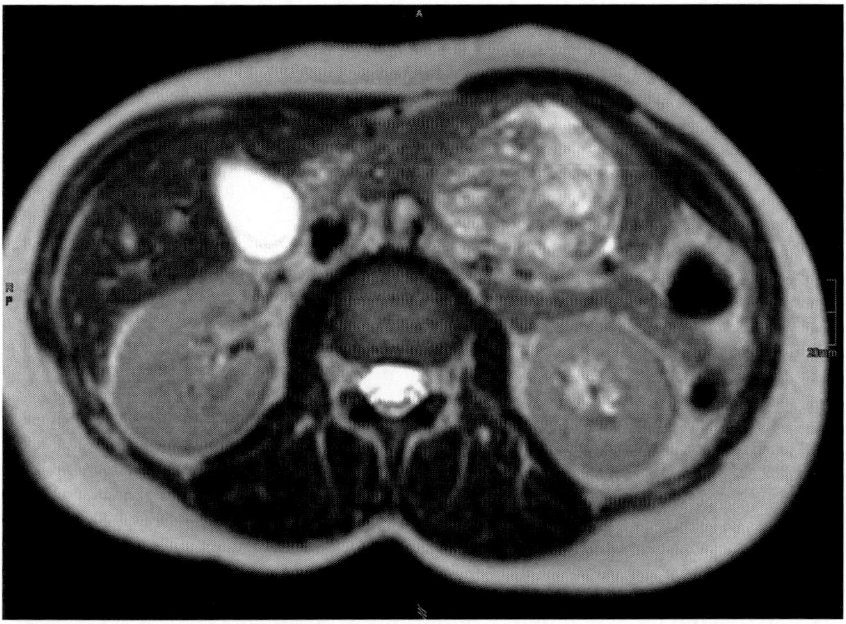

Figure 6. T2 weighted MRI image showing an inhomogenous, partially cystic lesion of the pancreatic tail – Undifferentiated carcinoma of the pancreas.

PET/CT AND PET/MRI

The hybrid imaging modalities PET/CT and PET/MRI, which combine functional PET imaging with CT or MRI, are presently not widely used for the differential diagnosis of cystic pancreatic lesions. Mainly, cystic pancreatic lesions are found as an incidental finding on PET/CT or PET/MRI performed for other reasons. The differential diagnosis of cystic pancreatic lesions on imaging depends on anatomical characteristics as described above, malignant signs like irregular wall thickening are often too small for detection on functional imaging, although there have been some studies which have shown that PET/CT might be helpful in the diagnosis of malignant cystic neoplasms or the differentiation of benign and malignant IPMNs. There is currently not enough data that would support the use of hybrid imaging in the management of cystic pancreatic lesions [15, 16, 17, 18].

Questions to Ask Regarding a Cystic Pancreatic Lesion

If a cystic lesion of the pancreas is detected on imaging the following imaging characteristics should be evaluated:

- How big is the lesion and where is it situated in the pancreas?
- Does the content of the lesion appear to be serous or are there areas which appear mucinous or solid?
- Is the cyst wall thin and regular or are there signs of wall thickening with nodular areas and, if applicable, contrast enhancement?
- If present, does contrast enhancement differ in the arterial and venous phase?
- Does the lesion contain calcifications or septae?
- Is it a singular lesion or are there more (cystic) lesions of the pancreas?
- Is the main pancreatic duct narrow or dilated? If dilatation is present, does it involve the whole pancreas or only parts of it?
- Is there communication of the lesion with the pancreatic duct system?
- Are there signs of chronic pancreatitis?

If a cystic lesion of the pancreas is detected on imaging the following patient characteristics should be evaluated:

- Gender and age of the patient?
- History of recurrent pancreatitis? History of malignancy?
- Signs of endocrine disease? History of genetic syndromes like MEN (multiple endocrine neoplasia) Type 1?
- Existence/Availability of previous imaging including ERCP?
- Relevant laboratory parameters (elevated lipase level, tumor markers etc.)?

Table 1. Imaging criteria of the most common cystic pancreatic lesions

	General imaging criteria
SCN	Usually solitary lesion, frequently in the pancreatic head Honeycomb appearance with mildly enhancing thin septae Occasionally visible central scar and/or calcifications No communication with pancreatic duct system
IPMN Branch duct type	Solitary or multiple lesions Grape-like cystic lesion with multiple enhancing septae Communication with pancreatic duct system Tanaka criteria: Worrisome features or high-risk stigmata possible [19]
IPMN Main duct type	Dilatation of the main pancreatic duct >10mm Usually no dilatation of bile duct Tanaka criteria: Worrisome features or high-risk stigmata possible
IPMN Mixed type	Combination of the above mentioned features
MCN	Solitary lesion, frequently in the pancreatic tail Thick, enhancing wall Frequently septae and nodules No communication with pancreatic duct
SPN	Solitary lesion Can be solid and/or cystic Calcifications and/or hemorrhage possible No communication with pancreatic duct
Pseudocyst	Solitary or multiple lesions Signs of (chronic) pancreatitis Thin, mildly enhancing to thick, enhancing cyst wall Simple serous cyst to complicated cysts filled with debris/signs of hemorrhage Communication with pancreatic duct possible Usually no or few septae
Rare cystic tumors	Multiple tumors can show cystic degeneration and mimic primary cystic pancreatic tumors: Neuroendocrine tumor – frequently strong enhancement of the cystic wall in the arterial phase Cystadenocarcinoma – no typical imaging criteria Undifferentiated Carcinoma – no typical imaging criteria Schwannoma – no typical imaging criteria Endometriosis – no typical imaging criteria

References

[1] Spinelli, K. S., Fromwiller T. E., Daniel R. A., et al. Cystic pancreatic neoplasms: observe or operate. *Ann. Surg*. 2004;239:651-9.

[2] Laffan, T. A., Horton, K. M., Klein, A. P., et al. Prevalence of unsuspected pancreatic cysts on MDCT. *AJR Am. J. Roentgenol.* 2008;191:802-7.

[3] Zhang, X. M., Mitchel, D. G., Dohke, M., Holland, G. A., Parker, L. Pancreatic cysts: depiction on single-shot fast spin-echo MR images. *Radiology* 2002;223:547-53.

[4] Adsay, N. V. Cystic neoplasia of the pancreas: pathology and biology. *J. Gastrointest. Surg.* 2008;12:401-4.

[5] Martin, R. C. G., Klimstra, D. S., Brennan, M. F., Conlon, K. C. "Solid-pseudopapillary tumor of the pancreas: a surgical enigma?" *Annals of Surgical Oncology* 2002;9(1);35–40.

[6] Kersting, S., Konopke, R., Kersting, F., Volk, A., Distler, M., Bergert, H., et al. Quantitative perfusion analysis of transabdominal contrast-enhanced ultrasonography of pancreatic masses and carcinomas. *Gastroenterology* 2009;137(6), 1903-1911.

[7] Richter, G. M., Simon, C., Hoffmann, V., DeBernardinis, M., Seelos, R., Senninger, N., Kauffmann, G. W. Hydrospiral CT of the pancreas in thin section technique. *Radiologe* 1996 May;36(5):397-405.

[8] Lee, H. J., Kim, M. J., Choi, J. Y., Hong, H. S., Kim, K. A. Relative accuracy of CT and MRI in the differentiation of benign from malignant pancreatic cystic lesions. *Clin. Radiol.* 2011; 66:315–321.

[9] Sahani, D. V., Sainani, N. I., Blake, M. A., Crippa, S., Mino-Kenudson, M., del-Castillo, C. F. Prospective evaluation of reader performance on MDCT in characterization of cystic pancreatic lesions and prediction of cyst biologic aggressiveness. *AJR* 2011; 197:72; [web]W53–W61.

[10] Sainani, N. I., Saokar, A., Deshpande, V., Fernandez-del Castillo, C., Hahn, P., Sahani, D. V. Comparative performance of MDCT and

MRI with MR cholangiopancreatography in characterizing small pancreatic cysts. *AJR* 2009; 193:722–731.

[11] Kawamoto, S., Lawler, L. P., Horton, K. M., Eng, J., Hruban, R. H., Fishman, E. K. MDCT of intraductal papillary mucinous neoplasm of the pancreas: evaluation of features predictive of invasive carcinoma. *AJR* 2006; 186:687–695.

[12] Procacci C, Carbognin G, Accordini S, et al. CT features of malignant mucinous cystic tumors of the pancreas. *Eur Radiol* 2001; 11:1626–1630.

[13] Visser, B. C., Yeh, B. M., Qayyum, A., Way, L. W., Mc-Culloch, C. E., Coakley, F. V. Characterization of cystic pancreatic masses: relative accuracy of CTand MRI. *AJR* 2007; 189:648–656.

[14] Lee, H. J., Kim, M. J., Choi, J. Y., Hong, H. S., Kim, K. A. Relative accuracy of CT and MRI in the differentiation of benign from malignant pancreatic cystic lesions. *Clin. Radiol*. 2011; 66:315–321.

[15] Sahani, D. V., Kambadakone, A., Macari, M., Takahashi, N., Chari, S., and Fernandez-del Castillo, C. Diagnosis and Management of Cystic Pancreatic Lesions. *American Journal of Roentgenology* 2013 200:2, 343-354.

[16] Tomimaru. Y., Takeda, Y., Tatsumi, M., et al. Utility of 2-[18F] fluoro-2-deoxy-D-glucose positron emission tomography in differential diagnosis of benign and malignant intraductal papillary-mucinous neoplasm of the pancreas. *Oncol. Rep*. 2010; 24:613–620.

[17] Mansour, J. C., Schwartz, L., Pandit-Taskar, N., et al. The utility of F-18 fluorodeoxyglucose whole body PET imaging for determining malignancy in cystic lesions of the pancreas. *J. Gastrointest. Surg.* 2006; 10:1354–1360.

[18] Sperti, C., Pasquali, C., Decet, G., Chierichetti, F., Liessi, G., Pedrazzoli, S. F-18-fluorodeoxyglucose positron emission tomography in differentiating malignant from benign pancreatic cysts: a prospective study. *J. Gastrointest. Surg.* 2005; 9:22–28; discussion, 28–29.

[19] Tanaka, M., Fernández-del Castillo, C., Adsay, V., et al. International consensus guidelines 2012 for the management of IPMN and MCN of the pancreas. *Pancreatology*. 2012;12(3):183-97.

In: Cystic Tumors of the Pancreas
Editor: Robert Grützmann
ISBN: 978-1-53612-523-8

Chapter 4

GASTROENTEROLOGICAL DIAGNOSIS

Roberto Valente*[1,2]*, MD, PhD,
Marco Del Chiaro*[1]*, MD, PhD, FACS
Miroslav Vujasinovic*[1]*, MD, PhD
Urban Arnelo*[1]*, MD, PhD
and Matthias Löhr*[1,*]*, MD, PhD
[1]CLINTEC - Karolinska University Hospital and Karolinska Institute, Stockholm, Sweden
[2]Digestive and Liver Disease Unit, Sapienza University of Rome, Italy

ABSTRACT

Pancreatic cancer is becoming a medical emergency and will be the second cause of cancer-related death by 2030. As has happened for other cancer types, such as colon and breast cancer, it is reasonable to assume that the main impact on disease management in the near future will involve the application of screening programs able to detect potential pre-neoplastic lesions, such as pancreatic cystic lesions, that are amenable to

* Corresponding Author Email: matthias.lohr@ki.se.

surgery. It is therefore crucial that, in addition to conventional radiology, we develop accurate gastroenterological diagnostic tools able to detect different types of lesions and to stratify the risk of possible malignancy.

Keywords: IPMN, Pancreatic cystic tumors, EUS, ERCP, pancreatoscopy, confocal laser endomicroscopy

INTRODUCTION

Pancreatic cancer is becoming a medical emergency [1] and, according to the World Health Organization (WHO), in 2030 it will probably be the second most common cause of cancer-related death [2]. It is also noteworthy that while for many tumors, including breast cancer, the mortality rate has declined over the last few decades; for pancreatic cancer it has remained stable or has moderately increased. In 2017, pancreatic cancer is expected to cause more deaths than breast cancer in the European Union (EU) [3]. The poor outcome related to this type of cancer is partly due to a lack of well-established screening programs for high risk individuals that would allow an effective early diagnosis and therapy for preneoplastic lesions [4].

Pancreatic cystic lesions (PCLs) display a prevalence of 20–30% in the general population [5, 6], of which 10-15% are pancreatic cystic neoplasms (PCNs). Of these, 21–33% are intraductal papillary mucinous neoplasms (IPMNs), which are considered to be precursor lesions for pancreatic cancer [7]. Although epidemiologically IPMNs have a major impact on the general population, their management is still hampered by a high rate of preoperative diagnostic error when evaluated with standard radiology, even in highly specialized third-level centers [8].

Since the potential therapeutic strategies for the management of IPMNs imply major surgical procedures such as pancreaticoduodenectomy and total pancreatectomy, which display considerable morbidity and mortality, an improvement in preoperative diagnostic accuracy is crucial.

Conventional cross-sectional imaging methods, such as magnetic resonance imaging (MRI) and computed tomography (CT) scanning, are widely available and provide a good overview of PCLs as well as the rest of the pancreas; nevertheless they are still hampered by a low diagnostic accuracy for the specific diagnosis of malignant lesions (44% and 44.7% for CT scans and MRI, respectively) [9]. Endoscopy, on the other hand, allows a full investigation of the main pancreatic duct (MPD) and, in addition to conventional cross-sectional radiology, it provides a complementary overview of the extent and nature of this complex disease.

Therefore, it is becoming evident that a single diagnostic strategy cannot be the solution to every problem. Furthermore, it is clear that the approach to such a complex disease should be supported by a multidisciplinary diagnostic work-up, including radiology and digestive endoscopy. This chapter provides a review of existing techniques and also a snapshot overview of possible future promising technologies that may help to identify patients at high risk of developing cancer [8].

Endoscopic Ultrasonography

Endoscopic ultrasound (EUS) involves combining endoscopy with high frequency ultrasound probes to allow a detailed exploration of the pancreas, a technique of diagnostic value in several pancreatic disorders including acute recurrent pancreatitis [10], chronic pancreatitis [11], and solid masses [12], as well as for the screening of individuals at high risk of developing pancreatic cancer [13] and the investigation of pancreatic cysts.

EUS is used in the diagnostic management of PCNs since it produces a high-resolution image offering a superb definition of the structural component of the cyst. There are currently two types of EUS probe: a radial probe that displays a 360° field of view [14], but does not permit the taking of histological samples, and a more recently developed linear probe, which allows tissue sampling through the operative channel. EUS also allows an accurate evaluation of cyst size, a careful description of its internal structural features and mural nodules as well as an assessment of a possible communication with the ductal system [15, 16], which is crucial for differential diagnosis.

Different types of cyst display specific ultrasound characteristics [9]; for example, serous cystadenoma (SCA), a microcystic, honeycomb-like cyst with a central stellate scar and no communication with the ductal system. In a minority of cases (10%), SCA displays a unilocular pattern with no clear microcystic component [17-21]. In contrast, mucinous cystadenoma (MCA) are usually multiloculated cysts with a visible wall on which eggshell calcifications may be present. These cysts can also show a granulated appearance mostly due to the presence of mucus, while intramural nodules, a solid component, and focal thickening of the cystic wall or septa suggest a possible malignancy [18, 20-22].

Table 1. Accuracy of EUS (EUS=Endoscopic Ultrasound; MRI = Magnetic Resonance Imaging; EUS-FNA = Endoscopic Ultrasound with Fine Needle Aspiration)

Authors	n	Study design	Outcome
de Jong, K., et al., Scand Journal Gastroenterol. 2012 [40]	32	Prospective cohort	Sensitivity and specificity: MRI (91% and 78%), respectively EUS (78% and 67%), respectively EUS-FNA (61% and 89%), respectively
Suzuki R., et al., Pancreatology. 2014 [29]	94	Meta analysis	EUS-FNA cytology for diagnosing malignant vs. benign IPMNs: Sensitivity - 64.8% Specificity - 90.6%.
Oppong K. W., et al., Pancreatology. 2015 [30]	133	Retrospective cohort	EUS diagnosis plus cytology plus intracystic CEA levels: Sensitivity - 91%, Specificity - 75% Accuracy - 85.7%
Wang, Q. X., et al., Cell Physiol Biochem. 2015 [58]	1024	Meta analysis	Pooled sensitivity and specificity for malignant EUS plus cytology: 51% and 94%, respectively Sensitivity and specificity for suspicious or potential malignancy EUS plus cytology: 52% and 97%, respectively
Hong, S. K., et al., Gastrointest Endosc 2012 [36]	66	Prospective cohort	EUS-FNA plus cystic wall puncture increases the diagnostic yield for mucinous or malignant cysts by around 29%. Adequate cytological sampling in 81% of patients

IPMN may appear as either a cyst or a cluster of cysts arising in the main pancreatic duct (PD) or its branches. IPMNs that exclusively involve the Wirsung duct are designated as main-duct IPMN (MD-IPMN), those involving the small branches are branch-duct IPMN (BD-IPMN), while those that involve both the main pancreatic duct and the peripheral branches are termed mixed-type IPMN [21]. The involvement of the main pancreatic duct can be either segmental or diffuse and is suspected preoperatively when the diameter of the Wirsung duct is >6 mm [5]. BD-IPMN can be either uni- or multifocal. From a diagnostic point of view, the most relevant feature in the differential diagnosis between IPMN and other cystic lesions is the presence of a communication with the pancreatic ductal system [9].

Pseudocysts are generally round, unilocular cystic lesions without internal septations or mural nodules. It is sometimes possible to identify mobile hyperechoic material inside the cyst, while the communication with the main pancreatic duct is often not observed [23]. Since pseudocysts are similar in appearance to other cystic lesions the diagnosis of a pseudocyst should not be given without having first carefully identified other signs of chronic pancreatitis in the rest of the pancreatic parenchyma.

Overall, EUS alone displays a high morphological resolution and a high detection rate; nevertheless, its accuracy in the differential diagnosis of PCNs is still far from 100%. In fact, Brugge et al. [24] reported only 56% sensitivity and 51% specificity when differentiating between mucinous versus non-mucinous cysts, with an overall low inter-observer agreement ($\kappa = 0.24$) for the differentiation of neoplastic versus non-neoplastic cysts [25]. Table 1 summarizes EUS accuracy.

EUS-FNA and Intracystic Fluid Markers

EUS-guided fine needle aspiration (EUS-FNA) allows the addition of cystic fluid analysis (biochemistry, viscosity, cytology and DNA analysis) to the morphological data, which improves the diagnostic yield. A large prospective multicenter study comparing the accuracy of EUS-FNA with carcinoembryonic antigen (CEA) measurement versus an EUS morphology assessment showed a 28% increase in diagnostic yield (79% vs. 51%, respectively) [24, 26]. In another series of 154 patients, when compared to CT and MRI, EUS-FNA increased the diagnostic yield of predicting a neoplastic cyst by 36% and 54%, respectively [27].

However, EUS-FNA should not be the sole solution to any diagnostic problem and the diagnostic accuracy of EUS-FNA for the differentiation of mucinous vs. non mucinous and malignant vs. non-malignant PCNs has been object of two recent meta-analyses. With respect to mucinous vs. non-mucinous PCNs, the pooled sensitivity and specificity were 63% and 88% respectively for CEA analysis and 54% and 93% for cytological analysis [28], while for malignant vs. non-malignant IPMNs, EUS-FNA-based cytology displayed a pooled sensitivity of 64.8% and a pooled specificity of 90.6% [29]. Oppong et al. evaluated a series of 133 patients undergoing EUS/EUS-FNA for suspected PCNs and found that while CEA, EUS, cytology and aspirate appearance displayed all a low accuracy (respectively 42.8%, 67.7%, 58.6% and 66.9%), combining the data provided a sensitivity of 91%, a specificity of 75% and an overall accuracy of 85.7% [30].

While CEA is considered to be the most accurate test for the presence of mucinous epithelia, it has certain shortcomings; for example, there is no definite cut-off although a multi-center prospective study reported that 192 ng/mL has an overall diagnostic accuracy of 79% for the detection of mucinous cysts [31, 32]. Additionally, CEA does not differentiate between IPMN and MCN, and does not correlate with the level of dysplasia or malignancy [33]; however, CEA levels seem most accurate at the extreme upper (>800 ng/mL for MCA) and lower (<5 ng/mL for SCA or pseudocysts) cut-off values [35].

Although CEA analysis has its limitations, cytological analysis also suffers from certain drawbacks, namely low cellularity in the aspirate and a limited volume of fluid available which restricts sensitivity to less than 50% [32]. In a prospective series of 144 patients, de Jong et al. reported adequate diagnostic material for cytological analysis in only 31% of patients and for biochemical analysis in 49% [34].

Another important factor for a successful diagnosis is cyst size – cysts should be >1.5 cm in order to obtain adequate material for analysis [25]. In addition, the application of rapid on-site evaluation (ROSE), as well as cyst wall puncture combined with CEA analysis appear to raise the diagnostic yield of EUS-FNA; however, results are still unclear and need further validation from wider studies [35, 36].

Overall, the complication rate for EUS-FNA on PCNs is between 2.2% and 6%. The great majority of complications include pancreatitis, hemorrhages and infections [37-39]. De Jong et al. compared the diagnostic value of MRI, EUS and EUS-FNA in differentiating between mucinous and non-mucinous PCNs and reported sensitivities of 61%, 78% and 91% respectively, suggesting a possible role for fine needle biopsy in increasing overall diagnostic accuracy [40].

Recently, Springer et al. used a previously described algorithm (MOCA) for analyzing multi-parametric features to identify markers capable of classifying cyst type and grade in a cohort of 130 patients with PCNs [41]. Fluid from each cyst was analyzed for subtle mutations in 6 oncogenes (BRAF, CTNNB1, GNAS, KRAS, NRAS, PI3K) and for mutations and loss of heterozygosity in 5 tumor suppressor genes (CDKN2A, RFN43, SMAD4 TP53, VHL), as well as the identification of aneuploidy. The group compared the accuracy of the molecular and clinical markers and a combination of molecular and clinical data and was able to classify the type of cyst with 90–100% sensitivity and 92–98% specificity. In addition, their panel of molecular markers was able to identify those patients who did not need surgery thus reducing the number of unnecessary interventions by 91% [41]. Table 2 summarizes the accuracy of EUS-FNA markers.

In conclusion, EUS (Figure 1) is a powerful even if potentially harmful diagnostic tool. Although its sensitivity and specificity are far from 100%, it can provide potentially useful diagnostic information in challenging PCL diagnoses in which the results are still unclear after conventional cross-sectional radiology [43].

Table 2. Accuracy of EUS-FNA Intracystic Markers (EUS = Endoscopic Ultrasound; CEA = Carcinoembryonic Antigen; CA19.9 = Carbohydrate Antigen 19.9)

Authors	n	Study design	Outcome
Brugge, W. R., et al., Gastroenterology 2004 [24]	341	Prospective multicenter	Accuracy CEA > 192 ng/mL = 79% Accuracy EUS morphology alone = 51% Accuracy cytology = 59%
van der Waaij, L. A., et al., Gastrointest Endosc. 2005 [59]	450	Pooled analysis	CEA > 800 ng/mL, suggestive for MCN CEA < 5 ng/mL or CA19.9 < 37 U/mL suggestive for Serous cystic Adenoma or Pseudocyst Amylase < 250 virtually excludes Pseudocyst Cytological sensitivity for malignancy = 48%
Thornton, G. D., et al., Pancreatology. 2013 [28]	1438	Meta analysis	Pooled sensitivities and specificities for cytology - 54% and 93%, respectively Pooled sensitivities and specificities for CEA intracystic levels - 63% and 88%, respectively
Kadayifci, A., et al. Dig Endosc. 2016 [60]	197	Retrospective cohort	GNAS + KRAS analysis on aspirate fluid collected by EUS-FNA increases diagnostic accuracy from 76.6% to 79.1% GNAS + CEA increases the diagnostic accuracy from 66.4% to 80.7% but no gain compared to KRAS alone. Triple combination analysis might improve yield to from single tests.
Gillis, A., et al. HPB (Oxford), 2015 [61]	362	Systematic review	Sensitivity and specificity of EUS-FNA cytology: 42% and 99% Sensitivity and specificity of KRAS analysis: 39% and 95% Sensitivity and specificity of KRAS plus Cytology: 71% and 88%

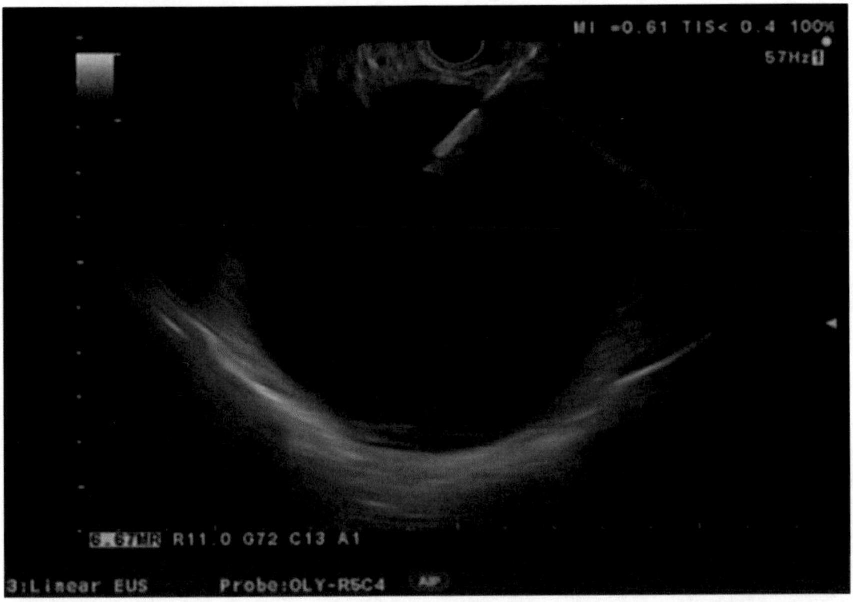

Figure 1. EUS-guided puncture of a pancreatic pseudocyst.

Endoscopic Retrograde Cholangiopancreatography (ERCP)

Endoscopic retrograde cholangiopancreatography (ERCP) now plays a limited role in PCL diagnosis. Both diagnostic cholangiography and pancreatography, once performed by ERCP, are now routinely carried out during magnetic resonance cholangiopancreatography (MRCP), which is less invasive and harmful, and the role of ERCP is generally exclusively therapeutic.

However, certain Japanese authors have suggested a possible diagnostic role for ERCP in patients with PCLs via analysis of biochemical markers in the collected pancreatic juice. In particular, Suzuki et al. performed a systematic review of 13 international studies with 483 IPMN patients to determine the diagnostic yield of cytology from ERCP. The authors reported a pooled sensitivity of 35.1% and specificity of 97.2% for distinguishing between benign and malignant IPMN [44]. Recently

Koshita et al. also investigated the possible role of pancreatic juice cytology (PJC) collected by ERCP and performed using the cell-block method (CB-PJC). The authors reported 50% sensitivity and 100% specificity for preoperative diagnosis of malignancy with only hematoxylin and eosin staining, and 79% sensitivity and 100% specificity by adding immunohistological staining [45].

Two typical endoscopic images consistent with the presence of IPMN are the "fish eye" sign (Figure 2) visualized during duodenoscopy, and an abnormal dilation of the main pancreatic duct seen on the pancreatogram (Figure 3).

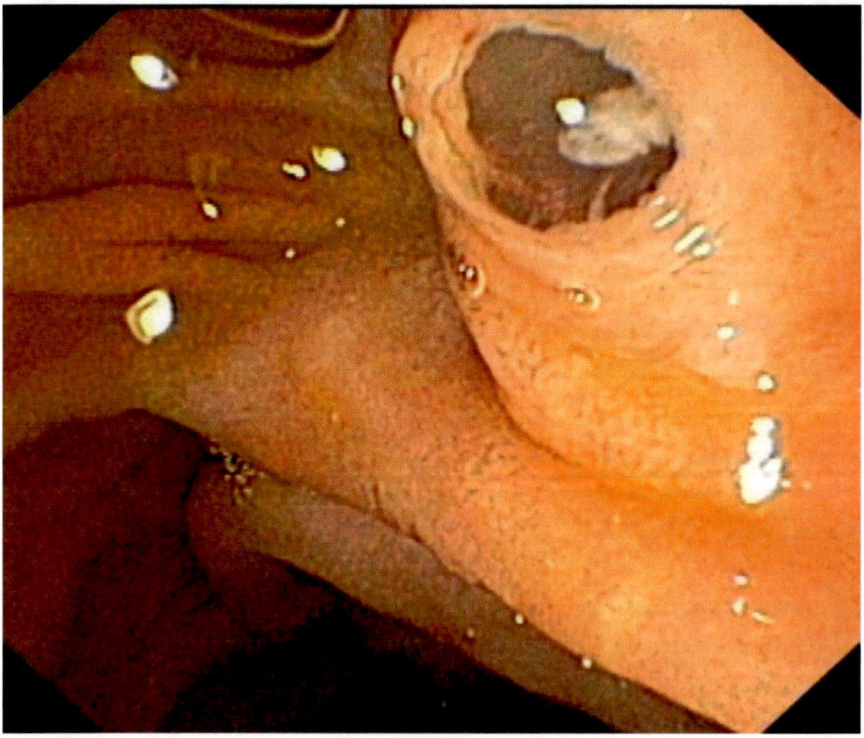

Figure 2. The "fish eye" sign visible during duodenoscopy for suspected IPMN.

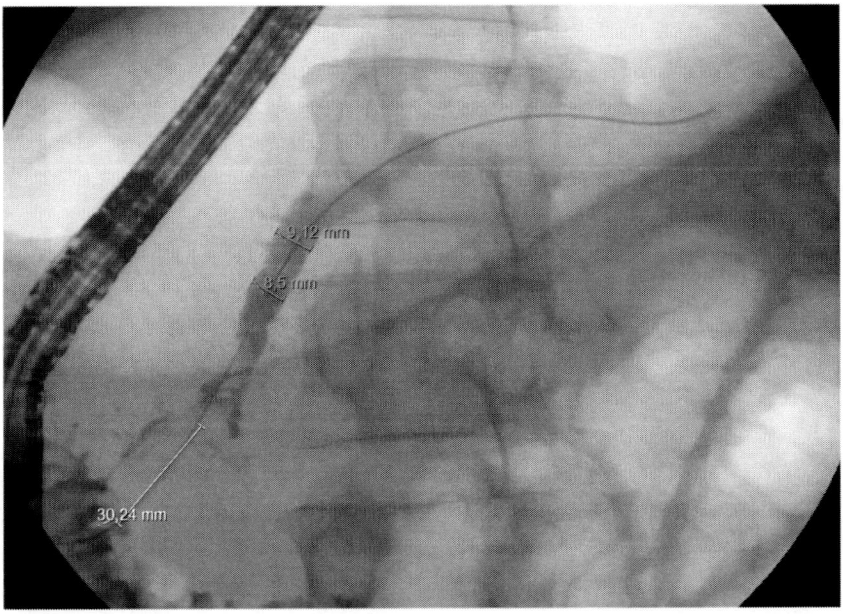

Figure 3. Pancreatogram showing abnormal dilation of the main pancreatic duct during ERCP.

In addition to its therapeutic applications, it is likely that ERCP will once again become a crucial diagnostic tool in the hands of endoscopists due to the development and wider application of new techniques, for example single operator cholangiopancreatoscopy (SOPC) and confocal laser endomicroscopy (CLE). These procedures allow a direct, microscopic view of the bile and pancreatic ducts and will probably become central to the investigation of pancreatico-biliary diseases, and in particular, diseases such as PCLs, in which the diagnostic accuracy is far from 100%.

PANCREATOSCOPY

Peroral intraductal endoscopy techniques for direct visualization of the biliary and pancreatic ducts were first described in the mid 1970's. However, technological challenges and procedural problems have meant that these procedures have not been used routinely [46].

Three cholangiopancreatoscopy techniques have been described so far: the oldest being a “dual-operator technique” that uses a mother-baby system and “direct” cholangioscopy, that employs an ultrathin transnasal gastroscope. Both provide good quality images with the possibility of applying narrow band imaging (NBI) to improve vascular definition; however, they have certain disadvantages: they are time consuming, difficult to maneuver, have a high incidence of complications, and the instruments are fragile and technically demanding to operate. Taken together, these features have strongly limited their routine use in clinical practice [46].

In 2007, the introduction of the first generation “single-operator” peroral cholangio-pancreatoscopy system (SpyGlass; Boston Scientific, Natick, Mass.) partially overcame these problems, by providing direct visualization of the biliary and pancreatic ducts with good quality images, improved maneuverability and no need for two endoscopists. This system has provided both diagnostic and therapeutic technological improvements, particularly in the management of biliary diseases, and overall has a low complication rate. More recently, a new digital cholangiopancreatoscopy system from Boston Scientific (Spyglass DS) has been introduced with several improvements, including image quality (6000 pixels) and resolution (Figure 4A and B). Technical characteristics for the various cholangiopancreatoscopy devices are shown in Table 3.

Irrespective of the probe used, the main applications of cholangiopancreatoscopy have so far been mostly limited to the investigation of the bile duct and there is little in the literature concerning pancreatic endoscopy compared to its biliary counterpart. This is probably due to an increased risk of complications, including post-ERCP pancreatitis that can reach up to 17% even in highly specialized centers [47]. In the “pre-Spyglass era,” the main studies available on the role of pancreatoscopy for the investigation of pancreatic neoplastic and pre-neoplastic lesions were performed using direct peroral mother-baby pancreatoscopy [49–51].

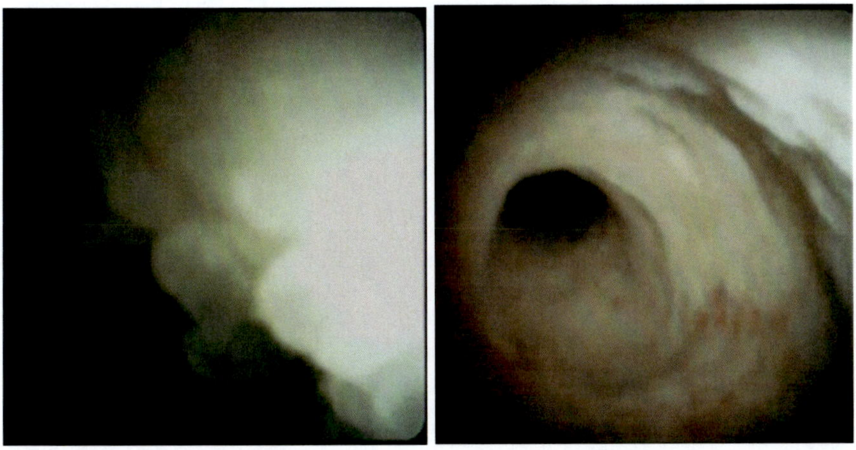

A B

Figure 4. Pancreatoscopy view with Spyglass of an IPMN (A) and abnormal upstream dilation of the main pancreatic duct (B).

In the "post-Spyglass era," Nagayoshi et al. investigated 17 patients with possible IPMN and MPD dilation using the Spyglass DS peroral pancreatoscopy system in 12 patients and an ERCP catheter in 5 patients. Targeted biopsies showed an overall low sensitivity (25%) but good specificity (100%) in detecting malignancy while the Spyglass system with irrigation cytology had 100% sensitivity and specificity for detecting malignancy [48].

Arnelo et al. published a prospective cohort-study of 44 consecutive patients with radiological diagnoses of IPMN who underwent Spyglass single-operator peroral pancreatoscopy. Their main aims were the diagnostic accuracy and possible complications of the procedure. The Spyglass procedure displayed an overall sensitivity of 84% and a specificity of 75%, providing additional diagnostic information in 95% of cases and showed the same accuracy as radiology in detecting MD-IPMN and greater accuracy in detecting BD-IPMN. In addition, as a complement to radiology, Spyglass pancreatoscopy changed the clinical decision making of multidisciplinary conferences in up to 76% of cases [47]. Table 4 compares and summarizes the diagnostic yields for the studies.

Table 3. Technical characteristics of available cholangiopancreatoscopic devices (Adapted from Tringali A., et al. Endoscopy, 2015)

Endoscope	Technology	Number of operators	Diameter (mm)	Working channel (mm)
CHF-BP30 (Olympus)	Fiber	Double	3.1	1.2 (single)
FCP-9P (Pentax)	Fiber	Double	3	1.15 (single)
CHF-B160 (Olympus)	Video	Double	4	1.2 (single)
CHF-B260 (Olympus)	Video	Double	3.4	1.2 (single)
CHF-B260 (Olympus)	Video	Double	2.6	0.5 (single)
Spyglass (Boston Scientific)	Video	Single	3.4	1.2 (multiple)
Spyglass DS (Boston Scientific)	Video	Single	3.3	1.2 (multiple)
PolyScope (PolyDiagnost)	Video	Double	2.7	1.2 (single)

Peroral pancreatoscopy can provide essential information regarding pancreatic disease, which helps to determine the extent of surgery required. In addition to its preoperative clinical diagnostic use, pancreatoscopy will also probably be employed in the near future as a complementary technique to facilitate the achievement of tumor-free margins during pancreaticoduodenectomy and to avoid missing skip lesions along the MPD during the resection of IPMNs [49]. Its main limitation is a possible risk related to the procedure itself that still need to be clarified and that demands further investigations in larger studies.

Table 4. Comparison of studies reporting pancreatoscopy for the investigation of IPMN (EUS = Endoscopic Ultrasound; IDUS= Intra-Ductal Endosonography)

Study	Year of publication	Technology used	Diagnostic Yield
Yamaguchi et al. [49]	2005	Mother-baby scope vs. catheter	Sensitivity of pancreatoscopy for pancreatic cytology vs. catheter (62.2% vs. 38.2%)
Hara et al. [50]	2002	Mother-baby scope vs. IDUS	Sensitivity of pancreatoscopy was 88% for MD-IPMN vs. 67% for BD-IPMN
Yasuda et al. [51]	2005	Mother-baby scope vs. IDUS and EUS	Detection rate of polyploid tumor >3 mm: 67%
Nagayoshi et al. [52]	2014	Spyglass	Sensitivity and specificity for targeted biopsies: 25% and 100%, respectively. Cytology sensitivity and specificity: both 100%
Arnelo et al. [48]	2014	Spyglass	Sensitivity: 84% Specificity: 75% Additional diagnostic information in 95% of cases

Confocal Laser Endomicroscopy (CLE)

CLE is another promising and potentially cost-effective new technique that can be applied to the management of PCNs. This technique has several possible future applications including improving the diagnostic yield in the cytological sampling of pancreatic lesions (when the cytologist is not on-site) and enhancing the differential diagnosis of mucinous vs. non-mucinous cystic lesions.

CLE is an innovative technology by which a single focal plane of tissue can be illuminated and scanned by a low power laser allowing the visualization of microscopic details (Figure 5). Three CLE systems have been developed: endoscope-based CLE (eCLE) that uses an integrated probe for upper and lower gastrointestinal (GI) investigations [50]; probe-based CLE (pCLE), which allows investigation of the bile duct and the pancreas and involves a separate CLE probe (Cellvizio; Mauna Kea Technologies Inc., Paris, France) that can be used with any endoscope [51]; and needle-based CLE (nCLE), specifically designed to access the target tissue by passing a mini-CLE probe (Cellvizio) through a 19-gauge needle during EUS-FNA to provide real-time imaging [52].

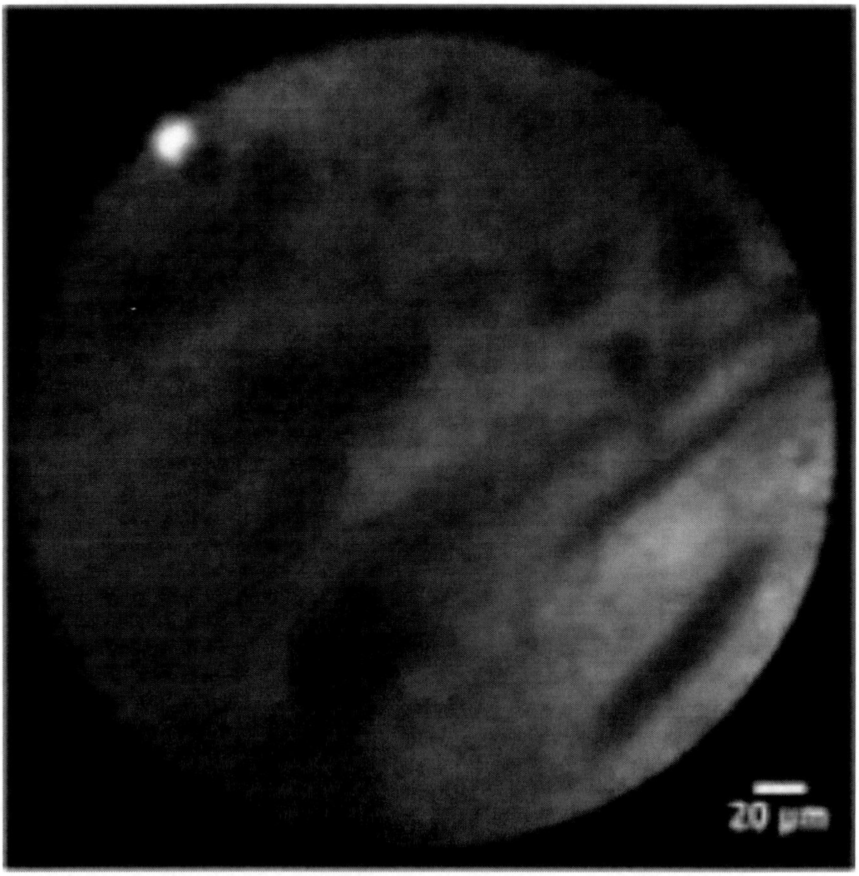

Figure 5. Confocal laser endomicroscopy showing a pattern consistent with pseudocyst.

In pCLE, the optical characteristics of the probe used determine the imaging depth (usually fixed) that can be reached [53]. The tip of the probe, placed in contact with the duct wall, delivers microscopic images while an intravenous injection of 10% fluorescein sodium (2.5–5.0 ml) provides contrast enhancement that lasts up to 45 min [54]. Two Cellvizio pCLE systems have been designed for use in intraductal biliopancreatic imaging:

The CholangioFlex miniprobe, which measures 0.96 mm in diameter; is compatible with the working channel of a cholangioscope, is radiopaque, provides 400-fold magnification, can reach a depth of 40–70 μm, and has a total field of view of 325×325 μm [51]. The GastroFlex probe is larger (diameter 2.6 mm) and used less often as it must be inserted freehand into the common bile duct (CBD), alongside a guidewire [51, 53].

Löhr et al. evaluated the application of pCLE together with mother-baby endoscopy (Spyglass) during ERCP in a series of 45 patients with IPMN and bile duct strictures in primary sclerosing cholangitis (PSC). The authors reported that the use of pCLE changed the diagnosis (based on histology and clinical follow-up) in 24 patients and had 91% sensitivity but only 52% specificity [51].

In summary, although a promising technique, pCLE requires further confirmation with regard to learning curve, diagnostic accuracy and reproducibility.

Needle-based CLE is the most recent of the three systems and has been widely investigated for the management of pancreatic cystic lesions. This technique has allowed the identification of new diagnostic criteria, including epithelial villous structures, which are associated with PCNs [55]; the presence of a superficial vascular network that is highly specific for the diagnosis of SCA [56]; a thick gray line (specific to MCN), a field of bright particles (pseudocysts), and black neoplastic cells clusters with white fibrous areas (cystic neuroendocrine neoplasm), amongst others [57].

In 2016, Krishna et al. evaluated the application of EUS-nCLE diagnostic criteria in a consecutive series of 49 patients surgically treated for PCLs; reporting overall sensitivity, specificity, and accuracy for diagnosing a mucinous PCL as 94%, 82%, and 89%, respectively, demonstrating that this technique improves the diagnostic accuracy of PCLs [52]. In conclusion, although these results are preliminary and have to be validated in larger prospective series, they seem to be very promising. Direct visualization and laser endomicroscopy evaluation of cystic lesions should have a deep impact in avoiding unnecessary surgery, allowing discrimination between mucinous and non-mucinous cystic neoplasms and providing a future basis for the development of a more cost-effective follow-up strategy.

REFERENCES

[1] Lohr JM. Pancreatic cancer should be treated as a medical emergency. *Bmj* 2014; 349: g5261.

[2] Rahib L, Smith BD, Aizenberg R et al. Projecting cancer incidence and deaths to 2030: the unexpected burden of thyroid, liver, and pancreas cancers in the United States. *Cancer Res* 2014; 74: 2913-2921.

[3] Ferlay J, Partensky C, Bray F. More deaths from pancreatic cancer than breast cancer in the EU by 2017. *Acta Oncol* 2016; 55: 1158-1160.

[4] Capurso G, Signoretti M, Valente R et al. Methods and outcomes of screening for pancreatic adenocarcinoma in high-risk individuals. *World J Gastrointest Endosc* 2015; 7: 833-842.

[5] Del Chiaro M, Verbeke C, Salvia R et al. European experts consensus statement on cystic tumours of the pancreas. *Dig Liver Dis* 2013; 45: 703-711.

[6] Del Chiaro M, Verbeke C. Cystic tumors of the pancreas: Opportunities and risks. *World J Gastrointest Pathophysiol* 2015; 6: 29-32.

[7] Del Chiaro M, Ateeb Z, Hansson MR et al. Survival Analysis and Risk for Progression of Intraductal Papillary Mucinous Neoplasia of the Pancreas (IPMN) Under Surveillance: A Single-Institution Experience. *Ann Surg Oncol* 2016.

[8] Del Chiaro M, Segersvard R, Pozzi Mucelli R et al. Comparison of preoperative conference-based diagnosis with histology of cystic tumors of the pancreas. *Ann Surg Oncol* 2014; 21: 1539-1544.

[9] But DY, Poley JW. To fine needle aspiration or not? An endosonographer's approach to pancreatic cystic lesions. *Endosc Ultrasound* 2014; 3: 82-90.

[10] Safari MT, Miri MB, Ebadi S et al. Comparing the Roles of EUS, ERCP and MRCP in Idiopathic Acute Recurrent Pancreatitis. *Clin Med Insights Gastroenterol* 2016; 9: 35-39.

[11] Petrone MC, Terracciano F, Perri F et al. Pancreatic abnormalities detected by endoscopic ultrasound (EUS) in patients without clinical signs of pancreatic disease: any difference between standard and Rosemont classification scoring? *Pancreatology* 2014; 14: 227-230.

[12] Saftoiu A, Vilmann P, Gorunescu F et al. Accuracy of endoscopic ultrasound elastography used for differential diagnosis of focal pancreatic masses: a multicenter study. *Endoscopy* 2011; 43: 596-603.

[13] Harinck F, Konings IC, Kluijt I et al. A multicentre comparative prospective blinded analysis of EUS and MRI for screening of pancreatic cancer in high-risk individuals. *Gut* 2016; 65: 1505-1513.

[14] Hass S AU, Löhr M, Iglesias-Garcia J. *Endoscopic Ultrasound (EUS) of Cystic Tumors of the Pancreas*. 2016; Cystic Tumors of the Pancreas.

[15] Lee KS, Sekhar A, Rofsky NM, Pedrosa I. Prevalence of incidental pancreatic cysts in the adult population on MR imaging. *Am J Gastroenterol* 2010; 105: 2079-2084.

[16] Jones MJ, Buchanan AS, Neal CP et al. Imaging of indeterminate pancreatic cystic lesions: a systematic review. *Pancreatology* 2013; 13: 436-442.

[17] O'Toole D, Palazzo L, Hammel P et al. Macrocystic pancreatic cystadenoma: The role of EUS and cyst fluid analysis in distinguishing mucinous and serous lesions. *Gastrointest Endosc* 2004; 59: 823-829.

[18] Kubo H, Nakamura K, Itaba S et al. Differential diagnosis of cystic tumors of the pancreas by endoscopic ultrasonography. *Endoscopy* 2009; 41: 684-689.

[19] Jais B, Rebours V, Malleo G et al. Serous cystic neoplasm of the pancreas: a multinational study of 2622 patients under the auspices of the International Association of Pancreatology and European Pancreatic Club *(European Study Group on Cystic Tumors of the Pancreas)*. 2016; 65: 305-312.

[20] Hruban RH KD, Pitman MB. *Atlas of Tumor Pathology*. 2006; Series IV. Washington (DC): Armed Forces Institute of Pathology.

[21] Hruban RH VC. Pathology and Classification of Cystic Tumors of the Pancreas. *Cystic Tumors of the Pancreas* 2016.

[22] Crippa S, Salvia R, Warshaw AL et al. Mucinous cystic neoplasm of the pancreas is not an aggressive entity: lessons from 163 resected patients. *Ann Surg* 2008; 247: 571-579.

[23] Bhosale P, Balachandran A, Tamm E. Imaging of benign and malignant cystic pancreatic lesions and a strategy for follow up. *World J Radiol* 2010; 2: 345-353.

[24] Brugge WR, Lewandrowski K, Lee-Lewandrowski E et al. Diagnosis of pancreatic cystic neoplasms: a report of the cooperative pancreatic cyst study. *Gastroenterology* 2004; 126: 1330-1336.

[25] Nakai Y, Isayama H, Itoi T et al. Role of endoscopic ultrasonography in pancreatic cystic neoplasms: where do we stand and where will we go? *Dig Endosc* 2014; 26: 135-143.

[26] Khalid A, Zahid M, Finkelstein SD et al. Pancreatic cyst fluid DNA analysis in evaluating pancreatic cysts: a report of the PANDA study. *Gastrointest Endosc* 2009; 69: 1095-1102.

[27] Khashab MA, Kim K, Lennon AM et al. Should we do EUS/FNA on patients with pancreatic cysts? The incremental diagnostic yield of EUS over CT/MRI for prediction of cystic neoplasms. *Pancreas* 2013; 42: 717-721.

[28] Thornton GD, McPhail MJ, Nayagam S et al. Endoscopic ultrasound guided fine needle aspiration for the diagnosis of pancreatic cystic neoplasms: a meta-analysis. *Pancreatology* 2013; 13: 48-57.

[29] Suzuki R, Thosani N, Annangi S et al. Diagnostic yield of EUS-FNA-based cytology distinguishing malignant and benign IPMNs: a systematic review and meta-analysis. *Pancreatology* 2014; 14: 380-384.

[30] Oppong KW, Dawwas MF, Charnley RM et al. EUS and EUS-FNA diagnosis of suspected pancreatic cystic neoplasms: Is the sum of the parts greater than the CEA? *Pancreatology* 2015; 15: 531-537.

[31] Stark A, Donahue TR, Reber HA, Hines OJ. Pancreatic Cyst Disease: A Review. *Jama* 2016; 315: 1882-1893.

[32] Oh HC, Kim MH, Hwang CY et al. Cystic lesions of the pancreas: challenging issues in clinical practice. *Am J Gastroenterol* 2008; 103: 229-239; quiz 228, 240.

[33] Maker AV, Carrara S, Jamieson NB et al. Cyst fluid biomarkers for intraductal papillary mucinous neoplasms of the pancreas: a critical review from the international expert meeting on pancreatic branch-duct-intraductal papillary mucinous neoplasms. *J Am Coll Surg* 2015; 220: 243-253.

[34] De Jong K, Poley JW, van Hooft JE et al. Endoscopic ultrasound-guided fine-needle aspiration of pancreatic cystic lesions provides inadequate material for cytology and laboratory analysis: initial results from a prospective study. *Endoscopy* 2011; 43: 585-590.

[35] Martin AK, Zhou Z. Endoscopic ultrasound-guided fine-needle aspiration for the diagnosis of pancreatic cysts by combined cytopathology and cystic content analysis. *World J Gastrointest* Endosc 2015; 7: 1157-1169.

[36] Hong SK, Loren DE, Rogart JN et al. Targeted cyst wall puncture and aspiration during EUS-FNA increases the diagnostic yield of premalignant and malignant pancreatic cysts. *Gastrointest Endosc* 2012; 75: 775-782.

[37] Tarantino I, Fabbri C, Di Mitri R et al. Complications of endoscopic ultrasound fine needle aspiration on pancreatic cystic lesions: final results from a large prospective multicenter study. *Dig Liver Dis* 2014; 46: 41-44.

[38] Lee LS, Saltzman JR, Bounds BC et al. EUS-guided fine needle aspiration of pancreatic cysts: a retrospective analysis of complications and their predictors. *Clin Gastroenterol Hepatol* 2005; 3: 231-236.

[39] Siddiqui AA, Shahid H, Shah A et al. High risk of acute pancreatitis after endoscopic ultrasound-guided fine needle aspiration of side branch intraductal papillary mucinous neoplasms. *Endosc Ultrasound* 2015; 4: 109-114.

[40] De Jong K, van Hooft JE, Nio CY et al. Accuracy of preoperative workup in a prospective series of surgically resected cystic pancreatic lesions. *Scand J Gastroenterol* 2012; 47: 1056-1063.

[41] Springer S, Wang Y, Dal Molin M et al. A combination of molecular markers and clinical features improve the classification of pancreatic cysts. *Gastroenterology* 2015; 149: 1501-1510.

[42] Radon TP, Massat NJ, Jones R et al. Identification of a Three-Biomarker Panel in Urine for Early Detection of Pancreatic Adenocarcinoma. *Clin Cancer Res* 2015; 21: 3512-3521.

[43] Marco del Chiaro UA, Roberto Valente. Letter to the Editor: Pancreatic cystic neoplasms: to needle or not to needle, this is the question. *American Journal of Gastroenterology* 2016 2016; accepted for publication.

[44] Suzuki R, Thosani N, Annangi S et al. Diagnostic yield of endoscopic retrograde cholangiopancreatography-based cytology for distinguishing malignant and benign intraductal papillary mucinous neoplasm: systematic review and meta-analysis. *Dig Endosc* 2014; 26: 586-593.

[45] Koshita S, Noda Y, Ito K et al. Pancreatic juice cytology with immunohistochemistry to detect malignancy and histological subtypes in patients with branch duct type intraductal papillary mucinous neoplasms of the pancreas. *Gastrointest Endosc* 2016.

[46] Judah JR, Draganov PV. Intraductal biliary and pancreatic endoscopy: an expanding scope of possibility. *World J Gastroenterol* 2008; 14: 3129-3136.

[47] Arnelo U, Siiki A, Swahn F et al. Single-operator pancreatoscopy is helpful in the evaluation of suspected intraductal papillary mucinous neoplasms (IPMN). *Pancreatology* 2014; 14: 510-514.

[48] Nagayoshi Y, Aso T, Ohtsuka T et al. Peroral pancreatoscopy using the SpyGlass system for the assessment of intraductal papillary mucinous neoplasm of the pancreas. *J Hepatobiliary Pancreat Sci* 2014; 21: 410-417.

[49] Tringali A, Lemmers A, Meves V et al. Intraductal biliopancreatic imaging: European Society of Gastrointestinal Endoscopy (ESGE) technology review. *Endoscopy* 2015; 47: 739-753.

[50] Goetz M, Watson A, Kiesslich R. Confocal laser endomicroscopy in gastrointestinal diseases. *J Biophotonics* 2011; 4: 498-508.

[51] Lohr JM, Lonnebro R, Stigliano S et al. Outcome of probe-based confocal laser endomicroscopy (pCLE) during endoscopic retrograde cholangiopancreatography: A single-center prospective study in 45 patients. *United European Gastroenterol J* 2015; 3: 551-560.

[52] Krishna SG, Swanson B, Hart PA et al. Validation of diagnostic characteristics of needle based confocal laser endomicroscopy in differentiation of pancreatic cystic lesions. *Endosc Int Open* 2016; 4: E1124-e1135.

[53] Konda VJ, Aslanian HR, Wallace MB et al. First assessment of needle-based confocal laser endomicroscopy during EUS-FNA procedures of the pancreas (with videos). *Gastrointest Endosc* 2011; 74: 1049-1060.

[54] Wallace MB, Meining A, Canto MI et al. The safety of intravenous fluorescein for confocal laser endomicroscopy in the gastrointestinal tract. *Aliment Pharmacol Ther* 2010; 31: 548-552.

[55] Konda VJ, Meining A, Jamil LH et al. A pilot study of in vivo identification of pancreatic cystic neoplasms with needle-based confocal laser endomicroscopy under endosonographic guidance. *Endoscopy* 2013; 45: 1006-1013.

[56] Napoleon B, Lemaistre AI, Pujol B et al. A novel approach to the diagnosis of pancreatic serous cystadenoma: needle-based confocal laser endomicroscopy. *Endoscopy* 2015; 47: 26-32.

[57] Napoleon B, Lemaistre AI, Pujol B et al. In vivo characterization of pancreatic cystic lesions by needle-based confocal laser endomicroscopy (nCLE): proposition of a comprehensive nCLE classification confirmed by an external retrospective evaluation. *Surg Endosc* 2015.

[58] Wang QX, Xiao J, Orange M et al. EUS-Guided FNA for Diagnosis of Pancreatic Cystic Lesions: a Meta-Analysis. *Cell Physiol Biochem* 2015; 36: 1197-1209.

[59] van der Waaij LA, van Dullemen HM, Porte RJ. Cyst fluid analysis in the differential diagnosis of pancreatic cystic lesions: a pooled analysis. *Gastrointest Endosc* 2005; 62: 383-389.

[60] Kadayifci A, Atar M, Wang JL et al. Value of adding GNAS testing to pancreatic cyst fluid KRAS and carcinoembryonic antigen analysis for the diagnosis of intraductal papillary mucinous neoplasms. *Dig Endosc* 2016.

[61] Gillis A, Cipollone I, Cousins G, Conlon K. Does EUS-FNA molecular analysis carry additional value when compared to cytology in the diagnosis of pancreatic cystic neoplasm? *A systematic review.* HPB (Oxford) 2015; 17: 377-386.

SECTION III. HISTOLOGY

In: Cystic Tumors of the Pancreas
Editor: Robert Grützmann
ISBN: 978-1-53612-523-8

Chapter 5

HISTOLOGY OF PANCREATIC CYSTIC TUMORS

Lena Häberle, MD and Irene Esposito*, MD, PhD
Institute of Pathology, Heinrich Heine University and University Hospital of Duesseldorf, Duesseldorf, Germany

ABSTRACT

As cystic lesions of the pancreas are increasingly diagnosed and resected, their characterization has advanced in the last few decades. The group now includes a large spectrum of heterogeneous entities, which can differ greatly in their biological behavior, making reliable differential diagnosis an important goal in order to ensure adequate patients' stratification. The clinically most relevant cystic lesions of the pancreas are true neoplasms, such as intraductal papillary mucinous neoplasms (IPMNs), mucinous cystic neoplasms (MCNs), serous cystic neoplasms (SCNs), cystic neuroendocrine tumors (cNETs) and solid pseudopapillary neoplasms (SPNs). These entities display distinct gross, histologic and immunophenotypic characteristics, and range from benign lesions to lesions with high risk of malignant transformation. In addition to the aforementioned lesions, rarer neoplastic epithelial lesions (e.g., cystic

* Corresponding Author Email: irene.esposito@med.uni-duesseldorf.de.

pancreatic ductal adenocarcinoma), neoplastic non-epithelial lesions (e.g., lymphangioma or cystic sarcoma), non-neoplastic epithelial lesions (e.g., congenital cysts) and non-neoplastic non-epithelial lesions (e.g., inflammatory pseudocysts) should also be considered in the differential diagnosis of pancreatic cysts.

Taking into account their distinct gross and histological features as well as their immunophenotypical characteristics is the key to an accurate diagnosis of cystic pancreatic tumors.

Keywords: Intraductal papillary mucinous neoplasm, IPMN, mucinous cystic neoplasm, MCN, serous cystic neoplasm, SCN, serous cystic adenoma, SCA, cystic neuroendocrine tumor, cNET, solid pseudopapillary lesion, SPN, pancreatic pseudocyst

INTRODUCTION

Cystic lesions of the pancreas are a heterogeneous group comprising a broad spectrum of entities, which are different in regard to their origin, biological behavior and prognosis. Accordingly, each entity displays distinctive morphologic features. The most common cystic pancreatic lesions are represented by a few neoplasms (namely, intraductal papillary mucinous neoplasms, IPMN; mucinous cystic neoplasms, MCN; serous cystic neoplasms, SCN; cystic neuroendocrine tumors, cNET and solid pseudopapillary neoplasms, SPN), mostly of epithelial origin, and by inflammatory pseudocysts. The nature of the cysts within this group is also heterogeneous and may result from increased mucin production and consequent duct dilatation, as in IPMN, or from hemorrhagic-necrotic degeneration, as in SPN. Inflammatory pseudocysts are devoid of an epithelial lining and are the result of reabsorption of necrotic debris after acute pancreatitis. As outlined in Table 1, dysontogenetic mechanisms, mechanical factors, such as duct obstruction, and even parasites may lie at the origin of pancreatic cystic lesions. Accurate gross and histopathological analysis is therefore of the utmost importance for the exact classification of cystic lesions of the pancreas, which then allows correct patients' stratification regarding clinical relevant issues, such as therapy, follow-up and prognosis.

In the following sections, the morphologic characteristics of the most common cystic neoplasms of the pancreas will be described in detail. An overview of the main morphological tools for differential diagnosis is presented in Table 3.

Table 1. Overview of cystic lesions of the pancreas. Modified from [1]

Neoplastic cystic lesions	**Non-Neoplastic cystic lesions**
Epithelial cystic lesions	
Intraductal papillary mucinous neoplasm (IPMN)	Congenital cyst
Mucinous cystic neoplasm (MCN)	Lymphoepithelial cyst
Serous cystic neoplasm (SCN)	Simple mucinous cyst
Serous cystadenoma, microcystic type	Enterogenic cyst
Serous cystadenoma,	Duodenal wall cyst
macrocystic/oligocystic type	Endometrial cyst
VHL-associated SCN Solid-type SCN (Serous cystadenocarcinoma)	Retention cyst
Cystic neuroendocrine tumor (cNET)	
Solid pseudopapillary neoplasm (SPN)	
Acinar cell cystadenoma	
Cystic acinar cell carcinoma	
Cystic pancreatic ductal adenocarcinoma	
Cystic pancreatoblastoma	
Cystic hamartoma	
Cystic teratoma	
Non-epithelial cystic lesions	
Lymphangioma	Pseudocyst (pancreatitis-associated)
Haemangioma	Parasitic cyst
Cystic sarcoma	

Intraductal Papillary Mucinous Neoplasms (IPMNs)

The group of intraductal papillary mucinous neoplasms (IPMNs) of the pancreas is heterogeneous in itself and consists of different macroscopic and microscopic subtypes.

IPMNs are mostly located in the pancreatic head. They are papillae-forming tumors that grow within the ducts of the pancreas and lead to a cystic dilation of the involved part of the pancreatic duct due to the production of varying amounts of mucins by the atypical epithelium. According to the current WHO definition, IPMNs are required to be more than 1 cm in diameter in order to distinguish them from pancreatic intraepithelial neoplasms (PanINs), which are usually smaller than 0.5 cm [2]. Lesions between 0.5 and 1 cm in diameter can be referred to as incipient IPMNs if they display other characteristics that are distinctive for IPMNs, such as the IPMN-typical mutation of GNAS codon 201 [3]. Macroscopically, IPMNs can be distinguished according to their localization in a main duct type, a branch duct type or a combined type: Main duct-type IPMNs show a distinct dilation of the main pancreatic duct, while branch duct-type IPMNs consist of one or more cysts in the pancreatic parenchyma that leave the main duct unaffected [4]. If main duct-type IPMNs extend to involve side branches of the pancreatic duct system as well or vice versa, they are considered combined-type IPMNs [5].

There are four distinct histological subtypes of IPMNs: The intestinal type, the pancreatobiliary type, the oncocytic type and the gastric type, each characterized by a distinct morphology of the papillary epithelium and a characteristic expression profile of immunohistochemical markers (Table 2) [6]. Main duct-type IPMNs are usually of the intestinal type or, less frequently, of the pancreatobiliary, oncocytic or gastric type, while branch duct-type IPMNs are usually of the gastric type [7].

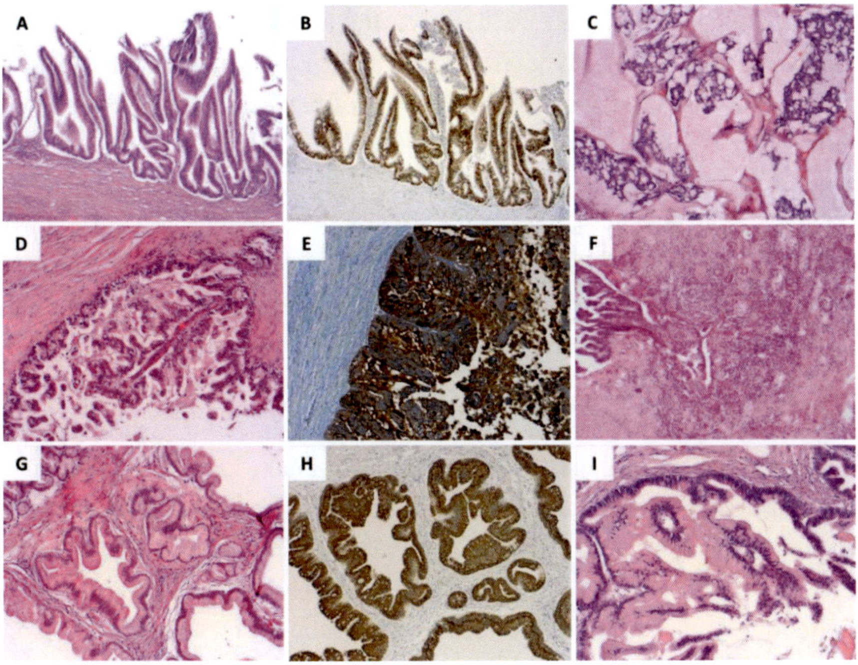

Figure 1. Histology of intraductal papillary mucinous neoplasms (IPMNs). **A.** IPMN of the intestinal type showing villous papillae. **B.** MUC2 positivity of intestinal-type IPMN in immunohistochemistry. **C.** Colloid carcinoma associated with intestinal-type IPMN showing pools of extracellular mucin. **D.** Pancreatobiliary-type IPMN displaying complex arborizing papillae. **E.** MUC1 positivity of pancreatobiliary-type IPMN in immunohistochemistry. **F.** Tubular (ductal) adenocarcinoma (upper half of picture) associated with pancreatobiliary-type IPMN (left). **G.** IPMN of the gastric type with foveolar papillae and abundant mucin in epithelial cells, low grade dysplasia. **H.** MUC5A positivity of gastric-type IPMN in immunohistochemistry. **I.** Gastric-type IPMN with high grade dysplasia.

Intestinal-type IPMNs display papillae that resemble villous adenoma of the colon. The epithelial cells are columnar with elongated nuclei and contain apical mucin. In immunohistochemistry, intestinal-type IPMNs are positive for the markers MUC2, MUC5A and CDX2, but negative for MUC1 [8] (Figure 1). In contrast, the papillae formed by pancreatobiliary-type IPMNs are more complex and branched. The epithelial cells are cuboidal with round nuclei and prominent nucleoli and contain less mucin compared to intestinal-type IPMNs. Pancreatobiliary-type IPMNs are positive for the markers MUC1 and MUC5A in immunohistochemistry, but are negative for MUC2 [8] (Figure 1). The appearance of oncocytic-type IPMNs is similar to pancreatobiliary-type IPMNs, hence they are viewed as a subtype of pancreatobiliary IPMNs by many authors. Their papillae also display a complex, arborizing architecture, which can contain solid and cribriform areas, but the cuboidal epithelial cells display a strikingly eosinophilic cytoplasm and round nuclei, often with a single prominent nucleolus. In immunohistochemistry, oncocytic-type IPMNs show a focal staining reaction for MUC1 and possibly of MUC2 (in goblet cells) and a diffuse staining reaction for MUC5A and MUC6 [8]. Gastric-type IPMNs form thicker and shorter papillae compared to the other IPMN types. The epithelium of gastric-type IPMNs resembles the gastric foveolar epithelium and the columnar epithelial cells contain abundant mucin. Immunohistochemically, gastric-type IPMNs are labelled by MUC5A, but are negative for MUC1 and MUC2 (Figure 1) [8].

As for all other precursor lesions of pancreatic ductal adenocarcinoma, the dysplasia in IPMNs should be classified as either high-grade or low-grade dysplasia according to their highest degree of dysplasia, with lesions formerly categorized as intermediate-grade dysplasia now belonging to the low-grade group [3].

All types of IPMNs can progress to invasive carcinoma. However, the malignant potential differs between the IPMN subtypes: in a Japanese multicentric study, gastric-type IPMNs only showed invasive carcinoma in 6.4% of the analysed cases, while oncocytic- and intestinal-type IPMNs had an associated invasive carcinoma in 25% and 34% of cases, respectively, and pancreatobiliary-type IPMNs showed an invasive component in 58% of cases (Table 2) [9]. The histological type of the IPMN-associated carcinoma also varies according to the IPMN subtype: intestinal-type IPMNs usually develop colloid carcinomas characterized by cancer cells in pools of extracellular mucin (Figure 1), while pancreatobiliary- and gastric-type IPMNs progress to tubular (classical ductal) carcinomas (Figure 1) and oncocytic-type IPMNs result in either tubular or oncocytic carcinomas (Table 2) [9].

Table 2. Overview of the subtypes of IPMNs

Histological type	Prevalence [9]	Localization	MUC1	MUC2	MUC5A	Other markers	Associated carcinoma
Intestinal	36%	Main duct	-	+	+	CDX2+	Colloid
Pancreatobiliary	6.7%	Main duct	+	-	+		Tubular
Oncocytic	8.5%	Main duct	Focal	Focal, goblet cells	+	MUC6+	Tubular, oncocytic
Gastric	49%	Branch duct	-	-	+		Tubular

Mucinous Cystic Neoplasms (MCNs)

Macroscopically, mucinous cystic neoplasms (MCNs) of the pancreas are large single cysts with thick, sometimes calcified walls. MCNs may be unilocular or multilocular. They usually show no communication with the pancreatic duct system, but may communicate with ducts in the case of fistulation [10]. The cyst fluid is typically mucinous, although contents may be more serous or hemorrhagic in some cases. Unlike IPMNs, MCNs are found almost exclusively in the distal pancreas [11].

MCNs consist of two characteristic histomorphological features: a columnar mucin-producing epithelium and an underlying ovarian-type stroma (Figure 2). This ovarian-type stroma consists of a large number of densely packed spindle-shaped cells and is entity-defining for MCNs [12, 13]. The ovarian-type stroma is thought to be derived either from ectopic ovarian tissue that is deposited in the pancreas during embryogenesis or from periductal fetal mesenchyme of the pancreas [14, 15]. Immunohistochemically, the epithelium of MCNs is labelled by MUC5A and CEA, while the ovarian-type stroma is characterized by the expression of estrogen and progesterone receptors as well as α-inhibin (Figure 2) [16, 17].

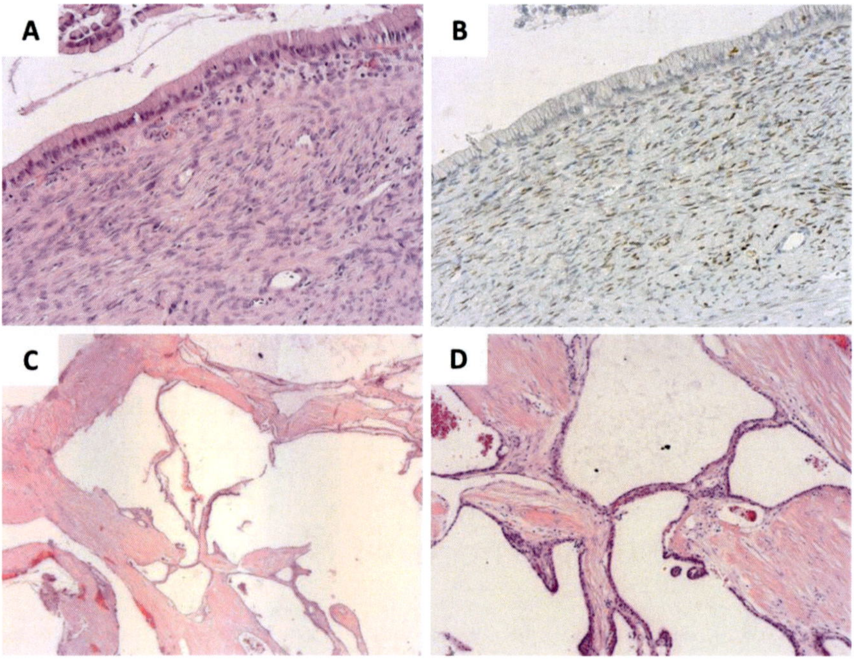

Figure 2. Histology of MCN and SCA. **A.** MCN displaying columnar mucin-producing epithelium and characteristic ovarian-type stroma. **B.** Expression of progesterone receptor by the ovarian-type stroma is shown in immunohistochemistry. **C.** SCA consists of multiple cysts separated by a collagen-rich stroma. **D.** The epithelium of SCA contains cuboidal cells with a clear cytoplasm and small, round nuclei.

The epithelial cells of MCNs can show a broad spectrum of dysplasia, even within a single lesion [11]. In analogy to IPMNs, MCNs should be classified as displaying low-grade or high-grade dysplasia according to the highest degree of dysplasia that can be observed in the lesion [3]. MCN epithelium can form papillae or mural nodules, which create intraluminal masses, usually indicating high-grade dysplasia or malignancy [11, 15]. However, only 4-20% of MCNs have an associated invasive carcinoma [10, 11, 13]. Invasive carcinoma arising in the context of MCN is usually of the tubular (classical ductal) type, although other rare types of have been described in association with MCNs (such as adenosquamous carcinoma, undifferentiated carcinoma with osteoclast-like giant cells, chorion-carcinoma and high-grade sarcoma [18-21]).

SEROUS CYSTIC NEOPLASMS (SCNS)

Serous cystic neoplasms (SCNs) of the pancreas include serous cystadenomas of the microcystic and macrocystic/oligocystic type as well as serous cystic neoplasms associated with Von Hippel Lindau syndrome (VHL). The solid-type SCN is an extremely rare variant. A malignant counterpart has been described in a number of case reports, but its existence has been recently debated [22].

Serous cystadenomas (SCAs) of the microcystic type are the most common form of SCNs (70-80% of the cases). Macroscopically, SCAs of the microcystic type are typically large, well-circumscribed single cysts. Upon cross-section, numerous small cysts filled with serous fluid (honeycomb or sponge-like appearance) and a central star-shaped scar, which may show calcification, are revealed. Like MCNs, SCAs of the microcystic type do not communicate with the pancreatic duct system and are often located in the pancreatic body or tail.

Macrocystic/oligocystic-type SCAs are rarer than their microcystic counterparts (20-25% of the cases). They have similar features as SCAs of the microcystic type, but contain fewer, but larger single cysts upon cross-section. They also lack the stellate scar usually displayed by SCAs of the microcystic type. According to a recent large series they are also more often found in the pancreatic body and tail [22].

VHL-associated SCNs generally share the same morphology as SCAs not associated with VHL syndrome; however, patients with VHL syndrome tend to have multiple SCNs involving the whole pancreas in a diffuse and sometimes patchy fashion [18].

Solid SCNs are extremely rare (<5%) and typically lack a central scar [22].

Microscopically, all SCNs display a cuboidal or flattened epithelium (Figure 2). The epithelial cells are characterized by a clear cytoplasm rich in glycogen and contain small, round hyperchromatic nuclei. The glycogen in the cytoplasm can be visualized using PAS stain. In immunohistochemistry, the expression of various cytokeratins, MUC1, MUC6, α-inhibin and neuron-specific enolase (NSE) by SCNs can be demonstrated [1]. Due to their expression of MUC1 and MUC6 it is presumed that SCNs could arise from centroacinar cells [1].

SCNs usually do not show dysplasia. Serous cystadenocarcinomas of the pancreas have been reported, but are exceedingly rare [22, 23].

CYSTIC NEUROENDOCRINE TUMORS (CNETS)

Neuroendocrine cystic tumors (cNETs) are a rare subgroup of pancreatic neuroendocrine tumors (NETs), which usually present as solid lesions. Macroscopically, cNETs are often unilocular, but may also be multilocular, and commonly contain a serous or hemorrhagic fluid [24, 25].

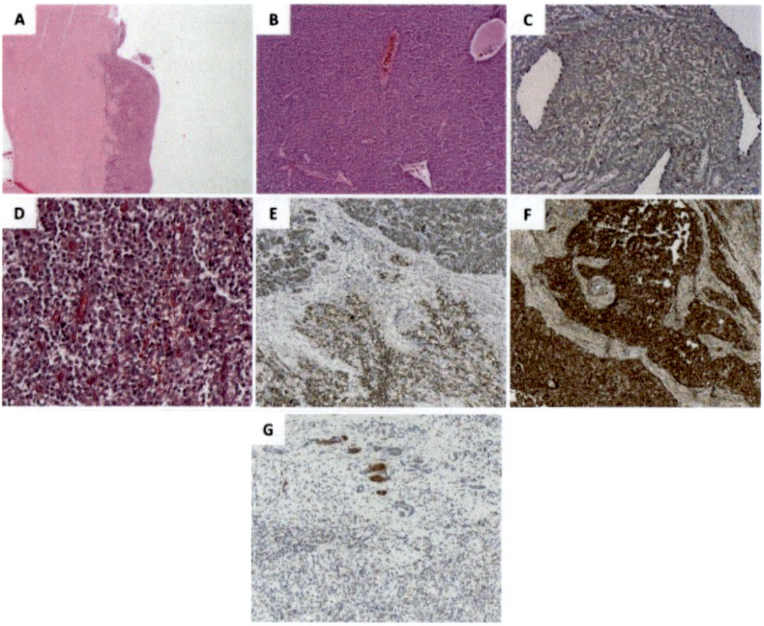

Figure 3. Histology of cNET and SPN. **A.** cNET comprised of cystic and solid areas. **B.** Solid areas of cNET show growth patterns typical for well-differentiated endocrine neoplasms of the pancreas. **C.** cNET with diffuse positivity for the neuroendocrine marker chromogranin A in immunohistochemistry. **D.** SPN displaying the typical monomorphic cells with eosinophilic cytoplasm and uniform nuclei, which can mimic neuroendocrine tumors. SPN stains positive for β-catenin (**E**), vimentin (**F**) and synaptophysin (**G**) at immunohistochemistry.

Histologically, cNETs are comprised of monotonous eosinophilic cells and may contain focal solid areas, in which the cells form trabecular patterns typical for well-differentiated endocrine neoplasms of the pancreas (Figure 3). It has been shown that cNETs often show a positivity for glucagon in immunohistochemistry [24].

SOLID PSEUDOPAPILLARY NEOPLASMS (SPNS)

Solid pseudopapillary neoplasms (SPNs) are large, well-circumscribed tumors that often present as cystic masses. However, SPNs do not contain true cysts, but rather caverns that are the result of a secondary degenerative process. On cross-section, SPNs may present either predominantly cystic or predominantly solid, depending on extent of necrosis the lesion underwent. Due to their origin, the cystic areas of SPNs can contain hemorrhagic or necrotic material.

In histology, SPNs contain solid areas contain clusters of relatively monotonous cells with an eosinophilic cytoplasm and uniform nuclei, which can mimic neuroendocrine tumors (NETs) (Figure 3). The clusters of cells are located around bands of stroma and small blood vessels. In less solid areas, the monomorphic cells form the eponymous pseudopapillary projections.

The cells of origin of SPNs are yet to be determined. SPNs show diffuse expression of vimentin, while staining for cytokeratins usually result in only focal or weak positivity [18]. In addition, they express CD10, progesterone receptor and commonly display nuclear positivity for beta-catenin (Figure 3). SPNs may express the neuroendocrine markers synaptophysin and neuron-specific enolase (NSE), but usually do not stain positive for chromogranin [18].

Table 3. Differential diagnosis of cystic neoplasms of the pancreas

Cystic lesion	Epidemiology	Localization	Macroscopic features	Histologic features	IHC
IPMN gastric type	M = F (50-70)	Head >> body of the pancreas	Involving pancreatic branch ducts	Thick short (foveolar) papillae	MUC1-, MUC2-, MUC5A+,
IPMN intestinal type			Involving pancreatic main duct	Long finger-like (villous) papillae	MUC1-, MUC2+, MUC5A+, CDX2+
IPMN pancreatobiliary type				Complex arborizing papillae	MUC1+, MUC2-, MUC5A+
IPMN oncocytic type				Complex arborizing papillae, eosinophilic cytoplasm	MUC1 focal, MUC2 focal/goblet cells, MUC5A+, MUC6+
MCN	F (40-60)	Tail of the pancreas	Single, thick-walled cyst, uni- or multilocular. No communication with duct system	Columnar mucin-producing epithelium, *ovarian-type* stroma	Epithelium: MUC5A+, CEA+; Stroma: estrogen and progesterone receptor+, α-inhibin+
SCA microcystic type	F > M	Body or tail of the pancreas	Multicystic *(honeycomb/ sponge-like)*, central star-shaped scar. No communication with duct system	Epithelial cells with clear cytoplasm, rich in glycogen	Cyto-keratins+, MUC1+, MUC6+, α-inhibin+, NSE+

Cystic lesion	Epidemiology	Localization	Macroscopic features	Histologic features	IHC
SCA macrocystic type	F > M	Body or tail of the pancreas	Multicystic (fewer, but larger cysts), no central scar. No communication with duct system	Epithelial cells with clear cytoplasm, rich in glycogen	Cyto-keratins+, MUC1+, MUC6+, α-inhibin+, NSE+
VHL-associated SCN	M = F	Whole pancreas, diffuse	No communication with duct system		
cNET		Whole pancreas	Uni- or multilocular. No communication with duct system	Uniform eosinophilic cells, trabecular growth	NET markers+, glucagon+
SPN	F >> M (10-30)	Whole pancreas	Caverns often with necrotic/ hemorrhagic material. No communication with duct system	Uniform eosinophilic cells, pseudo-papillae	Vimentin+, CD10+, proges-terone receptor+, β-catenin+ (nuclear), synaptophy-sin+, NSE+

REFERENCES

[1] Kosmahl, M., J. Wagner, K. Peters, B. Sipos, and G. Kloppel, Serous cystic neoplasms of the pancreas: an immunohistochemical analysis revealing alpha-inhibin, neuron-specific enolase, and MUC6 as new markers. *Am J Surg Pathol,* 2004. 28(3): p. 339-46.

[2] Adsay, N.V., Kloeppel, G., Fukushimam, N., et al., Intraductal Neoplasms of the Pancreas, in *WHO Classification of Tumors*, F.T. Bosman, Carneiro, F., Hruban, R.H., Theise, N.D., Editor. 2010, WHO Press: Lyon, France. p. 304-313.

[3] Basturk, O., S.M. Hong, L.D. Wood, et al., A Revised Classification System and Recommendations From the Baltimore Consensus Meeting for Neoplastic Precursor Lesions in the Pancreas. *Am J Surg Pathol,* 2015. 39(12): p. 1730-41.

[4] Tanaka, M., S. Chari, V. Adsay, et al., International consensus guidelines for management of intraductal papillary mucinous neoplasms and mucinous cystic neoplasms of the pancreas. *Pancreatology,* 2006. 6(1-2): p. 17-32.

[5] Salvia, R., S. Crippa, S. Partelli, et al., Differences between main-duct and branch-duct intraductal papillary mucinous neoplasms of the pancreas. *World Journal of Gastrointestinal Surgery,* 2010. **2**(10): p. 342-346.

[6] Furukawa, T., G. Kloppel, N. Volkan Adsay, et al., Classification of types of intraductal papillary-mucinous neoplasm of the pancreas: a consensus study. *Virchows Arch,* 2005. 447(5): p. 794-9.

[7] Ban, S., Y. Naitoh, M. Mino-Kenudson, et al., Intraductal papillary mucinous neoplasm (IPMN) of the pancreas: its histopathologic difference between 2 major types. *Am J Surg Pathol,* 2006. 30(12): p. 1561-9.

[8] Kloppel, G., O. Basturk, A.M. Schlitter, B. Konukiewitz, and I. Esposito, Intraductal neoplasms of the pancreas. *Semin Diagn Pathol,* 2014. 31(6): p. 452-66.

[9] Furukawa, T., T. Hatori, I. Fujita, et al., Prognostic relevance of morphological types of intraductal papillary mucinous neoplasms of the pancreas. *Gut,* 2011. 60(4): p. 509-516.

[10] Yamao, K., A. Yanagisawa, K. Takahashi, et al., Clinicopathological features and prognosis of mucinous cystic neoplasm with ovarian-type stroma: a multi-institutional study of the Japan pancreas society. *Pancreas,* 2011. 40(1): p. 67-71.

[11] Crippa, S., R. Salvia, A.L. Warshaw, et al., Mucinous cystic neoplasm of the pancreas is not an aggressive entity: lessons from 163 resected patients. *Ann Surg,* 2008. 247(4): p. 571-9.

[12] Takashima, M., T. Ueki, E. Nagai, et al., Carcinoma of the Ampulla of Vater Associated With or Without Adenoma: A Clinicopathologic Analysis of 198 Cases with Reference to p53 and Ki-67 Immunohistochemical Expressions. *Mod Pathol,* 2000. 13(12): p. 1300-1307.

[13] Goh, B.K., Y.M. Tan, Y.F. Chung, et al., A review of mucinous cystic neoplasms of the pancreas defined by ovarian-type stroma: clinicopathological features of 344 patients. *World J Surg*, 2006. 30(12): p. 2236-45.

[14] Volkan Adsay, N., Cystic lesions of the pancreas. *Mod Patho*l, 2007. 20 Suppl 1: p. S71-93.

[15] Zamboni, G., A. Scarpa, G. Bogina, et al., Mucinous cystic tumors of the pancreas: clinicopathological features, prognosis, and relationship to other mucinous cystic tumors. *Am J Surg Pathol,* 1999. 23(4): p. 410-22.

[16] Izumo, A., K. Yamaguchi, T. Eguchi, et al., Mucinous cystic tumor of the pancreas: immunohistochemical assessment of "ovarian-type stroma." *Oncol Rep*, 2003. 10(3): p. 515-25.

[17] Luttges, J., B. Feyerabend, T. Buchelt, M. Pacena, and G. Kloppel, The mucin profile of noninvasive and invasive mucinous cystic neoplasms of the pancreas. *Am J Surg Pathol,* 2002. 26(4): p. 466-71.

[18] Basturk, O., I. Coban, and N.V. Adsay, Pancreatic Cysts: Pathologic Classification, Differential Diagnosis, and Clinical Implications.

Archives of Pathology & Laboratory Medicine, 2009. 133(3): p. 423-438.

[19] Campman, S.C., M.A. Fajardo, M.B. Rippon, S.A. Kraegel, and B.H. Ruebner, Adenosquamous carcinoma arising in a mucinous cystadenoma of the pancreas. *J Surg Oncol,* 1997. 64(2): p. 159-62.

[20] Sarnaik, A.A., A.G. Saad, G.K. Mutema, S.P. Martin, A. Attar, and A.M. Lowy, Osteoclast-like giant cell tumor of the pancreas associated with a mucinous cystadenocarcinoma. *Surgery*, 2003. 133(6): p. 700-1.

[21] Wayne, M., D. Gur, G. Ascunce, B. Abodessa, and V. Ghali, Pancreatic mucinous cystic neoplasm with sarcomatous stroma metastasizing to liver: a case report and review of literature. *World Journal of Surgical Oncology,* 2013. 11: p. 100-100.

[22] Reid, M.D., H.J. Choi, B. Memis, et al., Serous Neoplasms of the Pancreas: A Clinicopathologic Analysis of 193 Cases and Literature Review With New Insights on Macrocystic and Solid Variants and Critical Reappraisal of So-called "Serous Cystadenocarcinoma." *Am J Surg Pathol,* 2015. 39(12): p. 1597-610.

[23] Jais, B., V. Rebours, G. Malleo, et al., Serous cystic neoplasm of the pancreas: a multinational study of 2622 patients under the auspices of the International Association of Pancreatology and European Pancreatic Club (European Study Group on Cystic Tumors of the Pancreas). *Gut,* 2016. 65(2): p. 305-12.

[24] Konukiewitz, B., T. Enosawa, and G. Kloppel, Glucagon expression in cystic pancreatic neuroendocrine neoplasms: an immune-histochemical analysis. *Virchows Arch,* 2011. 458(1): p. 47-53.

[25] Singhi, A.D., L.C. Chu, A.D. Tatsas, et al., Cystic pancreatic neuroendocrine tumors: a clinicopathologic study. *Am J Surg Pathol*, 2012. 36(11): p. 1666-73.

SECTION IV. MOLECULAR BACKGROUND

In: Cystic Tumors of the Pancreas
Editor: Robert Grützmann ISBN: 978-1-53612-523-8

Chapter 6

MOLECULAR BIOLOGY OF PANCREATIC CYSTIC TUMORS

Hai Yang and Christian Pilarsky*[*]*, MD, PhD
Department for Surgical Research, Universitätsklinikum Erlangen, Erlangen, Germany

ABSTRACT

Pancreatic cystic lesions (PCL) are divided into non-neoplastic and neoplastic. The neoplastic PCL are called pancreatic cystic tumors (PCT), mainly include serous cystic neoplasms (SCN), mucinous cystic neoplasms (MCN), intraductal neoplasms, solid pseudopapillary neoplasms (SPN) and others. With the development of medical imaging technology, the detection rate of PCTs increased yearly and the understanding of PCTs is also increasingly improved, but we still not fully understand the natural history and pathogenesis of PCTs. According to immunohistochemical and DNA sequencing analysis, each subtype of PCTs has its own specific changes. In most of SCN, MCN and intraductal neoplasms, the expression of epithelial markers are positive; the mutation of KRAS,TP53 and SMAD4 are more common in MCN and intraductal neoplasms; VHL signal pathway mutations may relate to SCN; Wnt / β-

[*] Corresponding Author Email: Christian.pilarsky@uk-erlangen.de.

catenin and Notch signaling pathways might play an important role in SPN. Understanding the molecular mechanism can help us to develop the method for early diagnosis and improve the treatment of PCTs.

Keywords: molecular background, cystic tumors, pancreas, kras, gnas

INTRODUCTION

Pancreatic cystic lesions (PCL) can be divided into non-neoplastic and neoplastic, with pancreatic pseudocysts as main type. Neoplastic PCLs main feature is that the cysts are formed by proliferation or ischesis of pancreatic duct or acinar epithelial cells. They can be mainly classified as serous cystic, mucinous cystic, intraductal and solid pseudopapillary neoplasms [1]. With the development of medical imaging technology, the detection rate of PCTs increased yearly. With the intense research of PCTs, numerous molecular markers have been used for the diagnosis of PCTs. Based on the common genetic changes of PCTs, the accuracy of diagnosis of PCTs can be improved by genetic diagnosis.

SEROUS CYSTIC NEOPLASMS

Serous cystic neoplasms (SCN) are usually cystic epithelial tumors that are composed of cuboidal and glycogen-rich epithelial cells, and can produce water-like serous liquid. Most of the SCN cases are benign, named serous cystadenoma. There are only a few cases of SCN that are malignant tumors, named serous cystdenocarcinoma [2].

The immunohistochemical expression of serous cystadenoma and its subtypes are indifferentiate. Because the epithelial characteristic, the immunohistochemical expression of serous cystadenoma shows that epithelial membrane antigens (EMA) CAM5.2, AE1/AE3 and cytokeratin (CK) 7,8,18,19 are positive [3, 4]. The expression of neuron-specific enolase (NSE) in serous cystadenoma is also positive, but the expression of other more specific markers of neuroendocrine differentiation, such as synaptophysin, chromogranin A (CgA) are negative [5, 6]. There is abnormal regulation in both disseminated and Von Hippel-Lindau (VHL) associated serous cystadenoma, expressing HIF-1a and CA IX [7].

In two VHL associated serous cystadenoma and 40-70% disseminated serous cystadenoma the loss of heterozygosity at the VHL gene locus was found [8]. Some case reports showed inactivation mutation of VHL gene in somatic cells of disseminated serous cystadenoma patients [9]. Unlike ductal adenocarcinomas, there is no KRAS and TP53 mutation in serous cystadenoma [3].

Mucinous Cystic Neoplasms

Pancreatic mucinous cystic neoplasms (MCN) are cystic epithelial tumors, and not connected to pancreatic duct system. The epithelial cells of MCN, which surrounded by ovarian-like stroma, are columnar epithelium and can produce mucilage. MCN is exclusively found in women. Depending on the grade of proliferation in epithelial cells of non-invasive MCN, it may be classified as MCN with low, moderate or severe dysplasia. Mucinous cystadenocarcinoma is MCN with invasive cancer components [1].

The epithelial markers, such as CK7, 8, 18, 19, EMA, carcino-embryonic antigen (CEA), are positive in MCN [10]. Gastrointestinal differentiation is also observed in MCNs [11]. The gastric type mucin marker MUC5AC and the pancreatic type mucin marker DUPAN-2, CA19-9 are positive expressed in neoplastic cells. Scattered goblet cells express MUC2 [12-14]. Most non-invasive MCN express SMAD4, but do not express MUC1. In contrast of non-invasive MCN, mucinous cystadenocarcinoma expresses MUC1 but lack of SMAD4 expression [15]. The ovary-like stroma which around epithelial cells express SMA, PR and ER [16].

The mutation in exon 12 of KRAS gene were found in both non-invasive MCN and mucinous cystadenocarcinoma, and this mutation increased in frequency with the grade of cell dysplasia [17]. Variation of tumor suppressor genes, such as TP53, CDKN2A and SMAD4, are much more common in mucinous cystadenocarcinoma. There are also CDKN2A abnormal methylation reported in some non-invasive MCN with low and moderate dysplasia [18].

Intraductal Neoplasms

Intraductal neoplasms includes intraductal papillary mucinous neoplasm (IPMN) and intraductal tubulopapillary neoplasms (ITPN). Intraductal neoplasms are primary and generally visible epithelial tumors in the pancreatic duct system, with differentiation of ductal epithelium. IPMN is overwhelmingly found in the main pancreatic duct and branch of pancreas. The tumor epithelium of IPMN are papillary, mucus-producing, and with different grades of epithelial dysplasia. Based on the highest grade of proliferation of cells and tissues, non-invasive IPMN can be classified as IPMN with low, moderate or severe dysplasia. Invasive IPMN with invasive cancer components is also known as intraductal papillary-mucinous carcinoma. Based on the location of pancreatic duct involvement, IPMN can be classified into main duct type, branch duct type and mixed duct type. IPMNs can also be subdivided into gastric-, intestinal-, pancreaticobiliary-, and oncocytic type according to their specific mucin expression [19, 20]. ITPN has small tubular structures with severe dysplasia, but without excessive mucus secretion. Intraductal tubulopapillary carcinoma is an ITPN with invasive cancer components.

CK7, CK19, B72.3 and CEA are strong positive in most IPMN. MUC1 is positively expressed in pancreaticobiliary-, and oncocytic type, but not in gastric-, and intestinal-type. MUC2 is only expressed in intestinal-type (Table 1) [21-23]. All components of cystic and low dysplasia in IPMN are pyloric gland, so they can express MUC6 [24]. Epidermal growth factor receptor is often expressed, and ERBB2 is often over-expressed [25]. With the grade of epithelial dysplasia increased, positive rate of Ki-67 coefficient and deletion expression ratio of CDKN2A are increased [26,

27]. There are p53 abnormal expression in a small number of high-grade IPMN, but not in low-grade IPMN [28]. Most IPMN express SMAD4, but there are higher deleted rate of SMAD4 in high-grade intraepithelial neoplasia and intraductal papillary-mucinous carcinoma [29]. The immunohistochemistry result of ITPN shows that ITPN comes from ductal epithelium. Expression of CK7, CK19 and PanCK are positive, but negative for the markers of acinar and endocrine [30]. The expression level of mucin is lower than mucinous adenocarcinoma and negative for MUC5AC and MUC2 [31, 32]. Most of the cases express SMAD4 [33].

Mutation rates of KRAS and GNAS between the different subtypes and localizations of IPMN differ only slightly, making these genes unsuitable as marker for the observed subtypes. The frequency of mutations in codons 12, 13 and 61 of KRAS in IPMN is 31%-86%. Recent studies suggest that the mutation rate may be around 50% [34]. This variability may be caused by the improvement in the definition and subclassification of IPMN [20]. Whole-exome sequencing showed that the mutation rate of GNAS in IPMN is 40%-60%, but not in pancreatic ductal adenocarcinoma [35, 36]. Gastric type and intestinal type have higher mutation rate of KRAS and GNAS than the other type of IPMNs (Table 2) [37, 38].

Table 1. Subtype classification and Immunohistochemistry expression of IPMN

	Subtype of IPMN			
	gastric	**intestinal**	**pancreaticobiliary**	**oncocytic**
MUC5AC	+	+	+	+
MUC1	-	-	+	+
MUC2	-	+	-	-
E-cadherin	+	+	+	+
β-catenin	+	+	+	+
CK7,19	+	+	+	+
B72.3	+	+	+	+
CEA	+	+	+	+

Table 2. Characteristics of KRAS and GNAS mutations in patients with IPMN

IPMN subtype	KRAS mutation	GNAS mutation
location of pancreatic duct		
main duct	61% (97/160)	56% (105/187)
branch duct	70% (191/272)	49% (160/327)
mixed duct	62% (58/94)	51% (45/89)
mucin expression		
Gastric	73% (228/314)	74% (122/164)
Pancreato biliary	72% (47/65)	53% (137/260)
Intestinal	44% (99/227)	24% (12/49)
Oncocytic	29% (5/17)	15% (2/13)

The allele deletion rate of some tumor suppressor genes such as CDKN2A, TP53 and SMAD4 can reach 40%, and is increased with the grade of epithelial dysplasia [39]. Although the mutation of CDKN2A is not so common, the lack of expression of CDKN2A caused by promoter methylation is much more common [40]. TP53 gene mutation showed in high-grade IPMN [41]. Allelic deletions at the SMAD4 locus are more common, but the SMAD4 gene mutation is very rare. Most non-invasive IPMNs express SMAD4 protein [33]. There are some cases reported that the mutations of STK11 happened in some patients with Peutz-Jeghers syndrome. This may suggest that STK11 mutations may contribute to sporadic IPMNs [42]. Taken together a precison medicine based classification system for IPMNs is still missing and the central marker for the genetic identifcation of subtypes have still to be discovered. However, GNAS mutations are the most important marker to delineate IPMNs from ductal adenocarcinoma and can be added to the arsenal of precision medicine for correct identifcation of IPMN cases.

SOLID PSEUDOPAPILLARY NEOPLASMS

Solid pseudopapillary neoplasms (SPN) are a low-grade malignancy, and occur in young women. SPN consists of morphologically identical epithelial cells with poor adhesion ability. Those cells form solid and pseudopapillary structures, often with bleeding and cystic degeneration [1].

The expressions of alpha-1-antitrypsin, alpha-2-antichymotrypsin, NSE, vimentin, progesterone receptors, CD10, CD56, claudin 5, galectin 3,cyclin D1 and cytoplasmic/nuclear β-catenin are all positive in nearly all SPNs [43-46]. SPNs have intense reaction to alpha-1-antitrypsin and alpha-2-antichymotrypsin, but this only happened in small cell clusters or single cells, and the distribution of positive cells is the same as eosinophilic globules NSE and vimentin often showed diffuse positive [43]. Immunohistochemically E-cadherin showed abnormal expression in the cytoplasmic and nuclear compartment [47]. The expressions of CgA, pancreatic hormones, ER-a, and AFP are negative in SPNs cells. Some cases showed positive expression of keratin [48-50].

The mutation of 3 exon of CTNNB1 gene which encodes β-catenin proteinis is found in somatic cells of almost all SPNs. This mutation results in the escape of intracellular phosphorylation in β-catenin, so that β-catenin will not be degraded. Then β-catenin can combine with Tef/Lef to form protein complex, this protein complex will be abnormally transported to the nucleus and activate the transcription of multiple oncogenes and cyclin D1, so that it will activate Wnt/β-catenin signal pathway. The activation of Wnt/β-catenin signal pathway can result in cell proliferation in other tumors, but the activation of cell proliferation in SPNs is not so high. This signal pathway may be blocked by the expression of p21 and p27 which the mechanism is still unknown [51]. The common molecular changes, such as KRAS, CDKN2A/p16, TP53 and SMAD4/DPC4, are not found in SPNs [52]. There is a study suggesting that the expression profile of SPNs is different from pancreatic ductal adenocarcinoma and pancreatic neuroendocrine tumors [43]. The main molecular changes are focused on the Wnt/β-catenin and Notch signaling pathways.

REFERENCES

[1] Bosman, F.T., World Health Organization., and International Agency for Research on Cancer, WHO classification of tumours of the digestive system. 4th ed. *World Health Organization classification of tumours.* 2010, Lyon: International Agency for Research on Cancer. 417 p.

[2] Perez-Ordonez, B., et al., Solid serous adenoma of the pancreas. The solid variant of serous cystadenoma? *Am J Surg Pathol,* 1996. 20(11): p. 1401-5.

[3] Ishikawa, T., et al., Immunohistochemical and molecular biological studies of serous cystadenoma of the pancreas. *Pancreas,* 1998. 16(1): p. 40-4.

[4] Santos, L.D., et al., Serous oligocystic adenoma of the pancreas: a clinicopathological and immunohistochemical study of three cases with ultrastructural findings. *Pathology,* 2002. 34(2): p. 148-56.

[5] Marsh, W.L., et al., Calponin is expressed in serous cystadenomas of the pancreas but not in adenocarcinomas or endocrine tumors. *Appl Immunohistochem Mol Morphol,* 2009. 17(3): p. 216-9.

[6] Oruc, N., et al., Cystic fluid chromogranin A levels in different pancreatic cystic lesions. *Turk J Gastroenterol,* 2015. 26(6): p. 522-7.

[7] Thirabanjasak, D., et al., Is serous cystadenoma of the pancreas a model of clear-cell-associated angiogenesis and tumorigenesis? *Pancreatology,* 2009. 9(1-2): p. 182-8.

[8] Vortmeyer, A.O., et al., Allelic deletion and mutation of the von Hippel-Lindau (VHL) tumor suppressor gene in pancreatic microcystic adenomas. *Am J Pathol,* 1997. 151(4): p. 951-6.

[9] Moore, P.S., et al., Molecular characterization of pancreatic serous microcystic adenomas: evidence for a tumor suppressor gene on chromosome 10q. *Am J Pathol,* 2001. 158(1): p. 317-21.

[10] Yamaguchi, K. and M. Enjoji, Cystic neoplasms of the pancreas. *Gastroenterology,* 1987. 92(6): p. 1934-43.

[11] Hayashi, H., et al., Hepatocellular carcinoma among hemodialysis patients infected with hepatitis C virus--early evolution and rapid progression. *Clin Nephrol,* 1999. 51(5): p. 321-3.

[12] Kosmahl, M., et al., Mucinous nonneoplastic cyst of the pancreas: a novel nonneoplastic cystic change? *Mod Pathol,* 2002. 15(2): p. 154-8.

[13] Sessa, F., et al., Ductal cancers of the pancreas frequently express markers of gastrointestinal epithelial cells. *Gastroenterology,* 1990. 98(6): p. 1655-65.

[14] Postlewait, L.M., et al., *Association of Preoperative Risk Factors With Malignancy in Pancreatic Mucinous Cystic Neoplasms: A Multicenter Study*. JAMA Surg, 2016.

[15] Kelly, P.J., et al., Cystic papillary pattern in pancreatic ductal adenocarcinoma: a heretofore undescribed morphologic pattern that mimics intraductal papillary mucinous carcinoma. *Am J Surg Pathol,* 2012. 36(5): p. 696-701.

[16] Qureshi, H.S., et al., Primary cutaneous mucinous carcinoma: presence of myoepithelial cells as a clue to the cutaneous origin. *Am J Dermatopathol,* 2004. 26(5): p. 353-8.

[17] Jimenez, R.E., et al., Sequential accumulation of K-ras mutations and p53 overexpression in the progression of pancreatic mucinous cystic neoplasms to malignancy. *Ann Surg,* 1999. 230(4): p. 501-9; discussion 509-11.

[18] Gerdes, B., et al., Tumor-suppressing pathways in cystic pancreatic tumors. *Pancreas, 2003*. 26(1): p. 42-8.

[19] Fong, Z.V. and C. Fernandez-Del Castillo, Intraductal Papillary Mucinous Neoplasm of the Pancreas. *Surg Clin North Am,* 2016. 96(6): p. 1431-1445.

[20] Grutzmann, R., et al., Intraductal papillary mucinous tumors of the pancreas: biology, diagnosis, and treatment. *Oncologist,* 2010. 15(12): p. 1294-309.

[21] Chang, X.Y., et al., [Intraductal tubulopapillary neoplasm of the pancreas: a clinicopathologic study of 6 cases]. *Zhonghua Bing Li Xue Za Zhi,* 2013. 42(4): p. 248-51.

[22] Toll, A.D. and M. Bibbo, Identification of gastrointestinal contamination in endoscopic ultrasound-guided pancreatic fine needle aspiration. *Acta Cytol,* 2010. 54(3): p. 245-8.

[23] Sclabas, G.M., et al., Frequency of subtypes of biliary intraductal papillary mucinous neoplasm and their MUC1, MUC2, and DPC4 expression patterns differ from pancreatic intraductal papillary mucinous neoplasm. *J Am Coll Surg,* 2012. 214(1): p. 27-32.

[24] Kobayashi, M., Y. Fujinaga, and H. Ota, Reappraisal of the Immunophenotype of Pancreatic Intraductal Papillary Mucinous Neoplasms (IPMNs)-Gastric Pyloric and Small Intestinal Immunophenotype Expression in Gastric and Intestinal Type IPMNs. *Acta Histochem Cytochem,* 2014. 47(2): p. 45-57.

[25] Schonleben, F., et al., Mutational analyses of multiple oncogenic pathways in intraductal papillary mucinous neoplasms of the pancreas. *Pancreas,* 2008. 36(2): p. 168-72.

[26] Mizumoto, M., et al., Molecular profile of apomucin and p53 protein as predictors of malignancy in intraductal papillary mucinous neoplasms of the pancreas. *Hepatogastroenterology,* 2011. 58(110-111): p. 1791-5.

[27] Yonezawa, S., et al., Precursor lesions of pancreatic cancer. *Gut Liver,* 2008. 2(3): p. 137-54.

[28] Tomaszewska, R., et al., HER-2/Neu expression as a progression marker in pancreatic intraepithelial neoplasia. *Pol J Pathol,* 1998. 49(2): p. 83-92.

[29] Ma, C., et al., Mutational spectrum of intraepithelial neoplasia in pancreatic heterotopia. *Hum Pathol,* 2016. 48: p. 117-21.

[30] Ahls, M.G., et al., Case report: Intraductal tubulopapillary neoplasm of the pancreas with unique clear cell phenotype. *Diagn Pathol,* 2014. 9: p. 11.

[31] Kolby, D., et al., Multifocal intraductal tubulopapillary neoplasm of the pancreas with total pancreatectomy: report of a case and review of literature. *Int J Clin Exp Pathol,* 2015. 8(8): p. 9672-80.

[32] Tajiri, T., et al., Diagnostic challenge: intraductal neoplasms of the pancreatobiliary system. *Pathol Res Pract,* 2012. 208(11): p. 691-6.

[33] Amato, E., et al., Targeted next-generation sequencing of cancer genes dissects the molecular profiles of intraductal papillary neoplasms of the pancreas. *J Pathol,* 2014. 233(3): p. 217-27.

[34] Schonleben, F., et al., BRAF and KRAS gene mutations in intraductal papillary mucinous neoplasm/carcinoma (IPMN/IPMC) of the pancreas. *Cancer Lett,* 2007. 249(2): p. 242-8.

[35] Furukawa, T., et al., Whole-exome sequencing uncovers frequent GNAS mutations in intraductal papillary mucinous neoplasms of the pancreas. *Sci Rep,* 2011. 1: p. 161.

[36] Wu, J., et al., Recurrent GNAS mutations define an unexpected pathway for pancreatic cyst development. *Sci Transl Med,* 2011. 3(92): p. 92ra66.

[37] Tan, M.C., et al., GNAS and KRAS Mutations Define Separate Progression Pathways in Intraductal Papillary Mucinous Neoplasm-Associated Carcinoma. *J Am Coll Surg,* 2015. 220(5): p. 845-54 e1.

[38] Lee, J.H., et al., KRAS, GNAS, and RNF43 mutations in intraductal papillary mucinous neoplasm of the pancreas: a meta-analysis. *Springerplus,* 2016. 5(1): p. 1172.

[39] Fujii, H., et al., Genetic progression and heterogeneity in intraductal papillary-mucinous neoplasms of the pancreas. *Am J Pathol,* 1997. 151(5): p. 1447-54.

[40] House, M.G., et al., Molecular progression of promoter methylation in intraductal papillary mucinous neoplasms (IPMN) of the pancreas. *Carcinogenesis,* 2003. 24(2): p. 193-8.

[41] Kanda, M., et al., Mutant TP53 in duodenal samples of pancreatic juice from patients with pancreatic cancer or high-grade dysplasia. *Clin Gastroenterol Hepatol,* 2013. 11(6): p. 719-30 e5.

[42] Su, G.H., et al., Germline and somatic mutations of the STK11/LKB1 Peutz-Jeghers gene in pancreatic and biliary cancers. *Am J Pathol,* 1999. 154(6): p. 1835-40.

[43] Aydiner, F., et al., Solid pseudopapillary tumor of the pancreas: emphasis on differential diagnosis from aggressive tumors of the pancreas. *Turk J Gastroenterol,* 2006. 17(3): p. 219-22.

[44] Raddaoui, E.M., et al., Differential diagnosis between pancreatic neuroendocrine and solid pseudopapillary neoplasms on endoscopic ultrasound-guided fine-needle aspiration. An immunohistochemical study. *Saudi Med J,* 2016. 37(7): p. 744-9.

[45] Comper, F., et al., Expression pattern of claudins 5 and 7 distinguishes solid-pseudopapillary from pancreatoblastoma, acinar cell and endocrine tumors of the pancreas. *Am J Surg Pathol,* 2009. 33(5): p. 768-74.

[46] Geers, C., et al., Solid and pseudopapillary tumor of the pancreas--review and new insights into pathogenesis. *Am J Surg Pathol,* 2006. 30(10): p. 1243-9.

[47] Kim, M.J., S.J. Jang, and E. Yu, Loss of E-cadherin and cytoplasmic-nuclear expression of beta-catenin are the most useful immunoprofiles in the diagnosis of solid-pseudopapillary neoplasm of the pancreas. *Hum Pathol,* 2008. 39(2): p. 251-8.

[48] Kloppel, G., et al., Solid-cystic (papillary-cystic) tumours within and outside the pancreas in men: report of two patients. *Virchows Arch A Pathol Anat Histopathol,* 1991. 418(2): p. 179-83.

[49] Miettinen, M., et al., Papillary cystic tumor of the pancreas. An analysis of cellular differentiation by electron microscopy and immunohistochemistry. *Am J Surg Pathol,* 1987. 11(11): p. 855-65.

[50] Nishihara, K., et al., Papillary cystic tumors of the pancreas. Assessment of their malignant potential. *Cancer,* 1993. 71(1): p. 82-92.

[51] Tiemann, K., et al., Solid pseudopapillary neoplasms of the pancreas show an interruption of the Wnt-signaling pathway and express gene products of 11q. *Mod Pathol,* 2007. 20(9): p. 955-60.

[52] Patel, S.A., et al., Genetic analysis of invasive carcinoma arising in intraductal oncocytic papillary neoplasm of the pancreas. *Am J Surg Pathol,* 2002. 26(8): p. 1071-7.

SECTION V. SURGERY

In: Cystic Tumors of the Pancreas
Editor: Robert Grützmann
ISBN: 978-1-53612-523-8

Chapter 7

SURGICAL PROCEDURES

Dimitrios Raptis*[*], *MD, Matthias Maak, MD, PhD and Robert Grützmann, MD, PhD, MBA
Department of Surgery, Friedrich-Alexander University of Erlangen-Nuremberg, Erlangen, Germany

ABSTRACT

Cystic tumors of the pancreas are more frequently diagnosed nowadays due to increased use of advanced imaging modalities. Treatement is most challenging and demands sometimes complex surgical approaches from skilled pancreatic surgeons in experienced, high-volume centers. The preferred surgical procedure depends on location, pathology of the cystic tumor, symptomatology, as well as infiltration of vessels or lymphnodes. Indicated procedures include pancreaticoduodenectomy – pylorus-sparing or Kausch-Whipple procedure -, left sided pancreatectomy, resection of the pancreatic corpus or the enucleation of benigne lesions in well-selected cases. Indication should always be discussed interdisciplinarily in tumor conferences, taking into consideration that these procedures are not always free of major complications.

Keywords: pancreatic cysts, cystic tumors of the pancreas, surgical approaches, surgical procedures

[*] Corresponding Author Email: dimitrios.raptis@uk-erlangen.de.

General Considerations

Cystic tumors of the pancreas represent a diagnostic and therapeutic challenge and nowadays are more commonly detected incidentally, by imaging for unrelated causes [1]. Given the malignant potential risk, surgeons, radiologists and gastroenterologists pay considerable attention to these cystic lesions and often the dilemma arrises, which approach, surgical resection or just surveillance, should be indicated.

As mentioned in previous chapters, cystic lesions of the pancreas are most detected incidentally and sometimes remain asymptomatic. In an epidemiologic study from Spinelli et al., 58% of patients diagnosed with a cystic tumor of the pancreas did not previously experience any episode of pancreatitis [2]. Although most patients undergo surveillance, surgical resection is indicated in cases of perceived or suspected malignancy and in patients with related symptoms.

Since 2013, exists a consensus statement from European experts, which provides guidelines for cystic tumors of the pancreas regarding their definition, classification, and diagnosis. Unfortunately prospective randomized trials are still lacking. Surgical approach is always indicated in all symptomatic cases and in cases with histological confirmed malignancy, in mucinous cystic neoplasm (MCN), solid pseudo-papillary neoplasm (SPN), main-duct intraductal papillary mucinous neoplasm (MD-IPMN), mixed-type IPMN, and in branch duct intraductal papillary mucinous neoplasm (BD-IPMN) when these lesions meet specific indications and resection-criteria [2, 3, 4].

Although specific considerations concerning diagnosis, treatment and follow-up for every cystic formation of the pancreas are mentioned and discussed in further detail in separate chapters of this book, it should be generally emphasized that in presence of malignancy or if malignancy can not be excluded, an oncological resection with lymphnode dissection should always be considered in patients fit for surgery.

The preferred surgical procedure depends on a) physical condition and the comorbidity of the patient, b) histopathological type of the cystic neoplasm, c) local extention of the tumor e.g., infiltration of pancreatic or biliary duct, vessel infiltration or infiltration of adjacent organs, d) presence of distant metastases, e) surgeon's experience, and f) patient's preference. Therapy should be individualized and the indication should always be discussed interdisciplinarily in tumor conferences. Surgical procedures should be performed only in high-volume centers, taking into consideration that pancreatic surgery is associated with a strong volume-outcome-relationship and mortality-rates are lower in well-experienced centers. For example unbiased mortality rates for pancreatic surgery procedures were determined using a comprehensive analysis of every inpatient case between 2009 and 2013 in a recent study in Germany. The overall in-hospital mortality rate (10.1%) did not significantly change during the study period. Major pancreatic resections were associated with mortality ranging from 7.3% (distal pancreatectomy) to 22.9% (total pancreatectomy). Overall in-hospital mortality rate was inversely associated with hospital volume quintiles, ranging from 6.1% in the very high volume quintile to 13% in the very low ones. After risk adjustment, the differences were slightly attenuated but statistically significant (11.5% vs. 6.5%) [5, 6].

SURGICAL PROCEDURES

Kausch-Whipple Partial Pancreaticoduodenectomy and Pylorus-Preserving Partial Pancreaticoduodenectomy (PPPD)

For cystic neoplasms located in or at the head of the pancreas a partial pancreatoduodenectomy should be considered. During this procedure the head of the pancreas with adherent duodenum including the ampulla of Vater, the gallblader, and the distal end of the bile duct are removed (view Figures 1, 1 A-E.

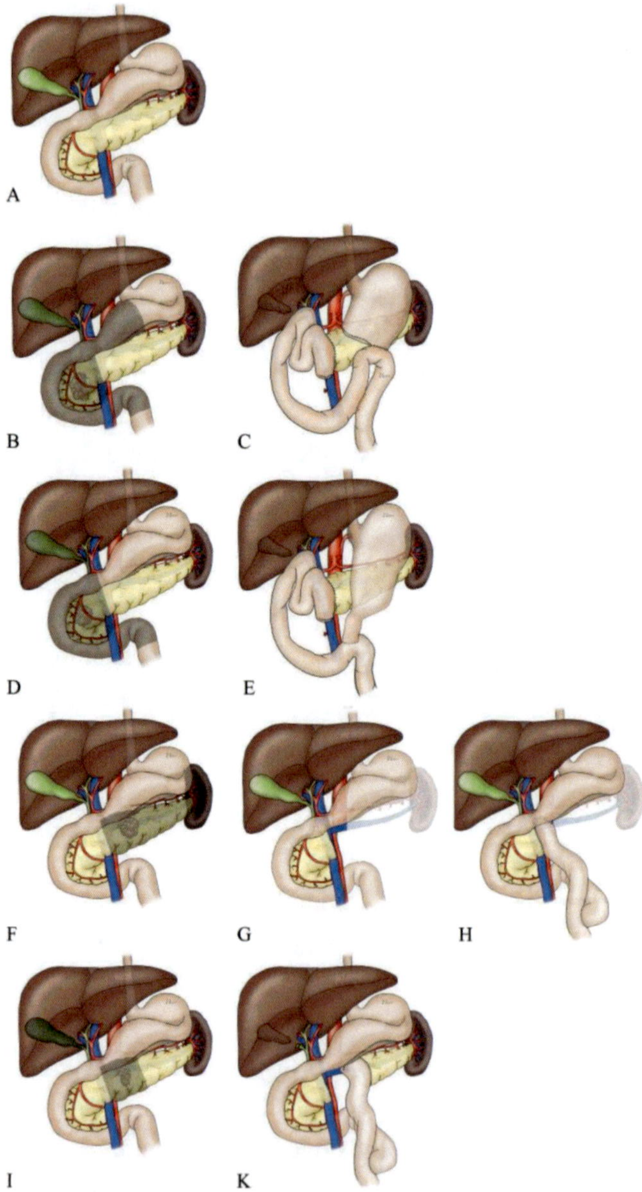

Figure 1. Illustrations of the operational procedures with the extent of the resection (shaded) and reconstruction. Shown are the normal anatomy (A), Kausch-Whipple procedure (B/C), PPPD (D/E), distal pancreatectomy with/without splenectomy and with /without pancreatojejunostomy(F/G/H) and middle segmental pancreatectomy (I/K).

The procedure typically begins with the exploration of the abdominal cavity, which always includes an ultrasonography of the liver to exlude a metastatic disease. Afterwards mobilization of the duodenum and the pancreatic head by the Kocher maneuver follows. An avascular plane can be achieved relatively easy. The posterior duodenal wall is mobilized. After the common hepatic artery is identified, the right gastric and pancreatoduodenal vessels are ligated and dissected. The gallblader is removed and the common bile duct dissected. Cholecystectomy is traditionally performed as part of the pancreaticoduodenectomy. The main reasons besides avoiding gallstone formation are the achievement of a wide and well-perfused hepatojejunostomy which can be better accomplished close to the bifurcation of the common bile duct, and an oncologically adequate lymphadenectomy. Further the second and third part of the duodenum is mobilized. The portal vein is located at the lower part of the pancreatic neck and is mobilized. Pancreatic veins that enter laterally into the portal vein are dissected after ligation. Mobilization continues with entering the lesser sac. The omentum gets lifted and dissected from transverse colon. In case of a Kausch-Whipple procedure the gastric antrum is transected using a stapler device. For a pylorus-preserving partial pancreaticoduodenectomy (PPPD) the first part of the duodenum is divided, also by using a stapler device. In our department, the head of the pancreas and the pancreatic duct are both routinely divided with a scalpel on a wooden chute in order to avoid thermal injury, stenosis or consequently anastomotic leakage and/or pancreatic fistula. The uncinate process gets isolated from the adjacent superior mesenteric vessels. The duodenal vessels get ligated. Margins are evaluated intraoperatively with routine frozen section after specimen removal. In case of margin infiltration with invasive carcinoma or high-grade dysplasia further resection in healthy margins is strictly recommended. A retrocolic reconstruction with one-loop is preferred. The pancreatojejunostomy is performed in two-layer interrupted way with 4x0 or 5x0 PDS-sutures. The hepatojejunostomy is carried out in one-layer manner with 4x0 PDS suture either continuous or interrupted depending on the surgeon and the size of the duct. Subsequently follows the duodenojejunostomy in one-layer continuous way with 4x0 PDS suture for the pylorus-preserving procedure or the gastrojejunostomy, in one-layer way (full-thickness and seromuscular) in cases of classic Whipple procedures.

In our surgical department we routinely perform the PPPD, in order to achieve a long-term improvement in gastrointestinal function, while the rates of delayed gastring empty (DGE) remain in an acceptable niveau. Furthermore PPPD shows comparable mortality, morbidity and oncological results compared with the classic Whipple operation [7]. Lymph node dissection is performed according to the latest European guidelines in cases of oncological resection.

Distal/Left Sided Pancreatectomy

For cystic tumors located in the pancreatic tail, a left sided pancreatectomy is considered. In many cases this can be carried out laparoscopically. Splenectomy is performed in cases of carcinoma, and/or nodal metastases in the splenic hilum, infiltration of spleen or splenic hilum or thrombosis/infiltration of the splenic vessels. An oncological resection of the tail of the pancreas always includes the appropriate lymph node dissection according to the latest guidelines (view Figures 1 F and G).

The procedure begins typically with the mobilization of the left colonic flexure from Gerota's fascia. The omentum majus then gets dissected from the transverse colon. The pancreas gets mobilized carefully from the transverse mesocolon. After splenic vessels are identified, mobilization of the medial pancreas is performed. Inspection of the pancreatic head and dissection of the left sided omentum majus is achieved with ligation of the short gastric arteries. Then ligation and dissection of the splenic vessels is carried out. In case of a laparoscopic procedure the pancreatic tail is dissected with an Endo-GIA device, in conventional left sided pancreatectomy with scalpel. In open procedures a fish-mouth reconstruction occasionally with falciform-ligament patch is preferred. A central stenosis of the main pancreatic duct should always be taken in consideration. In cases of its dilation at the resection site, a pancreatojejunostomy – mainly in means of Roux-en-Y- is indicated (view Figure 1 H).

Enucleation and Central or Middle Segmental Pancreatectomy

These parenchyma-preserving procedures are indicated only for benign or tumors with low-dysplasia, while they are strictly contraindicated for invasive cancers or tumors with suspicious malignant characteristica. Enucleation - laparoscopic or conventional - could be considered for small < 3cm, unifocal, and superficial lesions located commonly at the head of the pancreas or uncinate process, away from the main pancreatic duct [8, 9].

After enucleation, the main complication remains the development of pancreatic fistula. Incidence rates as high as 36.7% are reported [10]. For enucleation to be performed safely the lesion should be at least 2-3 mm from the main pancreatic duct and not too deep in the parenchyma. According to the published data from Crippa et al., grade B or C pancreatic fistulas are more common in patients with lesions of up to 2 cm in diameter, suggesting that the depth of the lesion in the parenchyma and its relationship to the pancreatic duct, rather than the size is closely associated with the incidence of pancreatic fistula [11]. After entering the lesser sac the partition of the pancreas carrying the lesion gets mobilized. An intraoperative ultrasonography is always performed to study the tumor morphology, to measure the distance to the main pancreatic duct, and to exclude the presence of a multifocal disease. The lesion is enucleated using scalpel during open procedure or coagulation device if performed laparoscopically. The specimen is always evaluated with frozen section to confirm clear margins or to proceed with subsequent re-resection. Enucleation should not be considered for an adequate oncological resection. According to an analysis from Turrini et al., enucleation for IPMN has less blood loss, shorter operative time, similar morbidity, mortality, hospital length stay and readmission rate, and should be considered more frequently as an option for unifocal BD-IPMNs < 3cm [12].

Central pancreatectomy (view Figures 1 I and K) is also a gland-sparing procedure, indicated for benign or lesions of "low-grade" malignancy, not suitable for enucleation, which are located at the pancreatic neck or body. Invasive carcinomas are an absolute contraindication for organ-sparing operations. Preventing a great loss of pancreatic parenchyma is a demanding challenge for the surgeon and could avoid insufficiency of the pancreatic function especially in fit patients with good prognosis [8, 9]. We usually perform this procedure in cases of neuroendocrine pancreatic lesions or for cystic tumors, when an invasive carcinoma has been excluded.

The procedure begins with the Kocher maneuver. The omentum gets lifted and dissected from the transverse colon. Consequently opening and entering of the lesser sac follows. Pancreatic gland gets mobilized from the superior mesenteric vein. Subsequently the splenic vein and its confluence into the superior mesenteric vein get identified. Small branches of the pancreas draining into splenic vein get ligated. The pancreatic specimen gets resected with safety margins. Extension of the resected gland depends on the localization and the histopathology of the tumor. The specimen routinely gets evaluated with frozen section to obtain the adequate resection margin. The caudal and cephalic sites of the remaining organ get controlled for hemostasis. At the central part of the pancreas the main duct gets sutured with 5x0 or 6x0 prolene; the parenchyma is sutured in fish-mouth technique. Concerning the anastomosis at the pancreatic tail we perform a retrocolic Roux-en-Y pancreato-jejunostomy (view Figure 1 K).

Concomitant Vascular Resections

Pancreatic tumors infiltrate commonly the portal vein or the superior mesenteric vein (mesenterico-portal axis). According to the latest guidelines an infiltration of these vessels, and especially of the portal vein, should not be a contraindication for an curative resection. Today in high-volume and well-experienced centers pancreatic tumors with vessel infiltration can be resected successfully in 20-30% of patients. A pancreas resection en-bloc with the infiltrated part of the vein is always indicated, when the tumor is adherent to the vein. Mortality and morbidity are not generally increased [13-16]. The type of venous resections vary between partial venous resection with direct closure (venorraphy), partial venous excision using a patch for the reconstruction, segmental resection with primary venous-venous anastomosis, tangential resection or segmental resection with interposed venous conduit and at least 2 anastomoses [13, 17, 18]. In our opinion the reconstruction with segmental resection is the most reliable method and can be performed in almost every case [17-19].

On the other hand in case of arterial infiltration a primary resection is usually contraindicated and is associated with increased mortality and morbididy rates [13-16]. Tumors of the pancreatic head most commonly infiltrate the superior mesenteric as well as the common hepatic artery. The splenic artery and the celiac axis are commonly infiltrated in cases of tumors located at the neck and tail of the pancreas.

In our opinion, and only in strictly selected cases, en bloc resection with curative intention could be performed. In cases of arterial infiltration, increased survival is reported for patients undergoing curative resection with en bloc arterial resection compared to patients treated only with palliative chemotherapy [19, 20]. An analysis from Johns Hopkins Hospital showed a significant difference in local recurrence rates (20 vs. 47%) but short-term survival was decreased significantly for patients who underwent an arterial resection [21]. Theoretically a total pancreatectomy could be a potential solution to avoid major complications after a high-risk arterial anastomosis complementing a pancreatectomy. After exclusion of inoperability with the "artery-first" maneuver, an arterial reconstruction could be performed with end-to-end or end-to-site primary anastomosis, in continous one-layer technique with Prolene-suture. Heparin flushing is strongly recommended after anastomosis is performed. As vascular graft could be used the splenic artery.

In cases of tumors of the pancreatic corpus or tail, infiltrating the celiac axis, an R0-resection without arterial reconstruction could be performed in selected cases. During this procedure – mostly known as "Appleby" Operation- pancreatic body and tail are resected en-bloc with the celiac axis and the spleen. An arterial reconstruction is not necessary and the perfussion of the liver remains retrogradely from the gastroduodenal artery via the superior mesenteric artery. Absolute contraindications are the infiltration of a) aorta, b) superior mesenteric artery, c) gastroduodenal artery, and d) proper hepatic artery [18-19].

It is strongly suggested that these procedures, and especially in cases of vessel infiltration should be limited to high-volume centers with multidisciplinary approach and experienced pancreatic surgeons with cross-collaboration opportunities, while not only visceral but also vascular surgical skills are necessary. Therapy should be individualized and the patient should be well-informed about the increased complication rates.

In cases of locally advanced, unresectable tumors, a multimodal concept with neo-adjuvant (radio-)chemotherapy should be considered. In a study from Erlangen and Oxford the numbers of infiltrated lymph nodes were decreased from 50% to 32% in patients with locally advanced pancreatic cancer who underwent neoadjuvant therapy. Moreover R0 resection was achieved in 95% of these patients with locally advanced pancreatic cancer [22]. In Germany, - under the leadership of the University Hospital of Erlangen- a multicentric, randomized study, also known as CONKO-007 study, is carried out. It compares chemo-radiation with chemotherapy alone after induction chemotherapy in patients with locally advanced, unresectable pancreatic tumors. First results will be published soon [23].

REFERENCES

[1] Scheiman, J. M. Cystic lesion of the pancreas. *Gastroenterology* 2005;128: 463–469.

[2] Spinelli, K. S., Fromwiller, T. E., Daniel, R. A., et al. Cystic pancreatic neoplasms: observe or operate. *Ann. Surg*. 2004; 239: 651–7.

[3] Del Chiaro, M., Verbeke, C., Salvia, R., et al. European Study Group on Cystic Tumours of the Pancreas. European experts' consensus statement on cystic tumours of the pancreas. *Dig. Liver Dis.* 2013; 45: 703-11.

[4] Kang, M. J., Jang, J. Y., Kim, S. J.,et al. Cyst growth rate predicts malignancy in patients with branch duct intraductal papillary mucinous neoplasms. *Clin. Gastroenterol. Hepatol.* 2011; 9: 87-93.

[5] Nimptsch, U., Krautz, C., Weber, G. F., Mansky, T, Grützmann, R. Nationwide In-hospital Mortality Following Pancreatic Surgery in Germany is Higher than Anticipated. *Ann. Surg.* 2016; 264: 1082-90.

[6] Krautz, C., Nimptsch, U., Weber, G. F., Mansky, T., Grützmann, R. Effect of Hospital Volume on In-hospital Morbidity and Mortality Following Pancreatic Surgery in Germany. *Ann. Surg.* 2017 Apr 4. [Epub ahead of print].

[7] Hüttner FJ, Fitzmaurice C, Schwarzer G, et al. Pylorus-preserving pancreaticoduodenectomy (pp Whipple) versus pancreaticoduodenectomy (classic Whipple) for surgical treatment of periampullary and pancreatic carcinoma. *Cochrane Database Syst Rev.* 2016; 2: CD006053.

[8] Zhi-Yong, Du., Shi Chen, Bao-San Han, et al. Middle segmental pancreatectomy: A safe and organ-preserving option for benign and low-grade malignant lesions. *World J. Gastroenterol.* 2013; 19: 1458-65.

[9] Iacono, C., Ruzzenente, A., Bortolasi, L., Guglielmi, A. Central pancreatectomy: The Dagradi Serio Iacono operation. Evolution of a surgical technique from the pioneers to the robotic approach. *World J. Gastroenterol.* 2014; 20: 15674-81.

[10] Beger, H. G., Siech, M., Poch, B., Mayer, B., Schoenberg, M. H. Limited surgery for benign tumours of the pancreas: a systematic review. *World J. Surg.* 2015; 39: 1557-66.

[11] Crippa, S., Bassi, C., Salvia, R., Falconi, M., Butturini, G., Pederzoli, P. Enucleation of pancreatic neoplasms. *Br. J. Surg.* 2007; 94: 1254-9.

[12] Turrini, O., Schmidt, C. M., Pitt, H. A., et al. Side-branch intraductal papillary mucinous neoplasms of the pancreatic head/uncinate: resection or enucleation? *HPB* (Oxford) 2011; 13: 126–31.

[13] Bockhorn, M., Uzunoglu, F. G., Adham, M., et al. Borderline resectable pancreatic cancer: a consensus statement by the International Study Group of Pancreatic Surgery (ISGPS). *Surgery.* 2014; 155: 977-88.

[14] *NCCN* Clinical Practice Guidelines in Oncology. Version 2. 2016.

[15] S3-*Leitlinien zum exokrinen Pankreaskarzinom*. Last accessed 20.12.2016.

[16] Ducreux, M., Cuhna, A. S., Caramella, C., et al. Cancer of the pancreas: ESMO Clinical Practice Guidelines for diagnosis, treatment and follow-up. *Ann. Oncol.* 2015;26 (suppl 5): 56-68.

[17] Grützmann, R., Kersting, S., Distler, Weitz J. Arterial reconstruction in pancreatic carcinoma-demonstration of surgical techniques *Zentralbl. Chir*. 2014; 139: 261-4.

[18] Grützmann, R., Distler, M., Weitz, J. Appleby operation for locally advanced tumour of the pancreatic body and tail—a video demonstration. *Zentralbl. Chir*. 2015; 140: 151-4.

[19] Raptis, D., Maak, M., Gruetzmann, R. *CHAZ*. 17. Jahrgang 4. Heft. 2016.

[20] Mollberg, N., Rahbari, N. N., Koch, M., et al. Arterial resection during pancreatectomy for pancreatic cancer: a systematic review and metaanalysis. *Ann. Surg.* 2011; 254: 882-93.

[21] Glebova, N., Hicks, C. W., Tosoian, J. J., et al. Outcomes of arterial resection during pancreatectomy for tumor. *J. Vasc. Surg*. 2016; 63: 722-29.

[22] Tinkl, D., Grabendauer, G. G., Golcher, H., et al. Downstaging of pancreatic carcinoma after neoadjuvant chemoradiation. *Strahlenther Onkol.* 2009; 185: 557-66.

[23] Pancreatic carcinoma: chemoradiation compared with chemotherapy alone after induction chemotherapy (CONKO-007). *Clinical Trials.gov Identifier*: NCT01827553. https//clinicaltrials.gov/ct2/show/NCT01827553.

Section VI. Diagnostic and Therapeutic Particularities of Specific Tumor Entities

In: Cystic Tumors of the Pancreas
Editor: Robert Grützmann
ISBN: 978-1-53612-523-8

Chapter 8

SEROUS CYSTIC NEOPLASMS OF THE PANCREAS

Emrullah Birgin, MD and Felix Rückert*, MD, PhD
Surgical Department, University Hospital Mannheim,
Mannheim, Germany

ABSTRACT

Serous cystic neoplasms (SCNs) belong to the benign cystic lesions of the pancreas. Due to the high number of medical imaging, this type of lesion is increasingly diagnosed. Histologically, all types of SCNs are determined by flattened glycogen-rich serous cells. A malignant transformation is a very rare event, so SCNs are defined as benign lesions. Symptomatic lesions are rare, and the gold standard in terms of diagnosis is an MRI and CT scan. A surgical approach should only be performed if the SCN is symptomatic or if there is the suspicion of malignancy. The present chapter gives a comprehensive overview over important characteristics of this entity and is interesting for clinicians with a focus on the pancreas.

* Corresponding Author Email: felix.rueckert@umm.de.

Keywords: serous cystic neoplasm, pancreatic cystic neoplasms, serous microcystic adenoma, serous oligocystic adenoma, von hippel-lindau disease

Introduction

Serous cystic neoplasms (SCN) represent an important entity among the cystic lesions of the pancreas. SCNs have to be distinguished from BD-IPMN [1, 2]. SCNs were first described by Compagno et al. in 1978 [3]. Some confusion resulted from inconsistent nomenclature. In the past, "glycogen-rich cystadenomas" and "serous cystadenoma" were expressions used equally for SCNs (e.g., [4]). Recently, more evidence was added (e.g., [5, 6]), and the present chapter highlights current knowledge concerning this entity, which is frequently seen by clinicians. After summarizing facts on the pathophysiology, we will go into detail on clinical characteristics, diagnostic, treatment and prognosis of SCN.

Pathophysiology of SCN

Cystic lesions of the pancreas are structured by means of different classification systems. The WHO classification and the third series of the Armed Forces Institute of Pathology (AFIP) fascicle subdivides these lesions on the basis of their histological type and biological behavior into benign tumors, borderline and malignant tumors [7]. The majority of the SCN is benign, although very rare reports about malignant transformation exist.

Cystic lesions can further be subdivided into peripheral, which do not communicate with the main pancreatic duct, and ductal tumors according to their site of origin [4]. SCN clearly belong to the peripheral tumors. According to Kosmahl et al. cystic processes within the pancreas can also be sorted by a simple two step classification system. In a first step cysts are classified into neoplastic and non-neoplastic cysts. In a second step, the cysts are separated into those with and without an epithelial lining. This classification then results in four groups: neoplastic epithelial or non-epithelial and non-neoplastic epithelial or non-epithelial [8]. Using this system SCN are non-neoplastic epithelial cysts. The synopsis of previous reports showed no distinct favorite localization of SCN within the pancreas [5, 6, 9]. SCN can therefore be seen in every part of the pancreas. Pancreatic duct communication is only seen in the smallest part of SCN (0.6%) [9] (Figures 1 A and B).

Microscopically, SCN are defined by the presence of a single layer of cuboidal or flattened glycogen-rich serous cells lining the small cysts. Their cells are negative for mucin stains, and the glycogen can be highlighted by PAS stain [10]. The cells have well-defined cytoplasmic borders, pale to clear cytoplasm, and small, round uniform nuclei with dense, homogeneous chromatin and inconspicuous nucleoli. The nuclear contours are very smooth. Atypia and mitosis are absent. The cuboid cells are intimately admixed with prominent capillary network [11, 12]. SCN might assumably arise from the centroacinar cell/intercalated duct system [13]. A study by Kosmahl et al. showed that NSE, α-inhibin, and MUC6 are markers for SCN [11]. The cuboid cells also express cytokeratins AE1/AE3, CAM 5.2, CK7, CK8, CK18 and CK19 while most other MUCs are negative [11, 12]. Staining for β-catenin also suggested a membranous reaction [13].

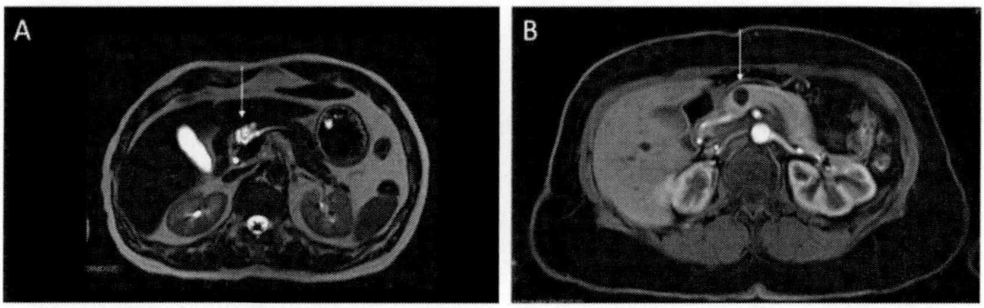

Figure 1. MRI scan of cystic lesions which were later histologically diagnosed as microcystic (A) and macrocystic (B) SCN. White arrows indicate the lesions.

The cuboidal cells of the cysts do not harbor the typical genetic fingerprint of pancreatic cancer or mucinous preneoplasias, namely Kras, SMADH4/DPC4, p53, and $p16^{Ink}$ genes [10]. However, gene alterations detected in the pathogenesis of von Hippel-Lindau disease (VHL) might play a role as gene alterations like loss of heterozygosity at chromosome 3p25 and a VHL-gene germline mutation are detected in 40% of the cases [8, 14]. Interestingly, Glut-1, a molecule involved in glycogen metabolism, is also expressed consistently in serous tumors [10].

Macroscopically, the cut surface of SCN shows numerous, tightly packed, small, thin-walled cysts resembling a spongelike appearance. These cysts are arranged around a central stellate scar, which may contain calcifications [8]. The central stellate scar and the stroma separating the cysts are composed of acellular collagenous connective tissue [12].

The group of SCN encompasses different macroscopic forms, and recently it was proposed to divide these into four types [6, 11, 15] (Figure 2). The first is the microcystic type of SCN (also "serous microcystic adenoma" (SMA)). The second is the macrocystic type of SCN (probably corresponding to "serous oligocystic and ill-demarcated adenoma" (SOIA)). The third is the mixed microcystic and macrocystic type and the last is the solid type [11, 15]. To the group of SCN also belong the von Hippel Lindau-associated cystic neoplasms and the serous cystadenocarcinoma, which can show the above mentioned macroscopic types and are composed of the same cell type (12). Macrocystic types show cysts $\geq$ 2mm and lack the central scar. This variant occurs predominantly in the head of the pancreas (8). Mixed microcystic and macrocystic types are defined by a combination of a microcystic and macrocystic pattern. Solid SCN is a tumor without cystic lesions distinguishable on cross-sectional imaging [6, 15].

Solid tumors consist of the above mentioned cuboidal cells and stain immunohistochemically for α-inhibin and are negative for Vimentin. Cystic calcifications are present in 15% [6]. The frequency of microcystic type is 45%, of macrocystic type 32%, of the mixed micro-and macrocystic type 18% and for the solid type 5% [6].

It is controversial discussed, if SCN might show a malignant transformation. Malignant SCN- the so called serous cystadenocarcinomas- seem to be a rarity. SCN is defined to be malignant if "distant metastasis beyond the peripancreatic bed" occur [6, 16]. Only few malignant SCN have been described [6, 15]. Microscopically, these carcinomas are identical to SCN. No morphologic findings other than behavior have been found to distinguish these malignant variants from their benign counterparts. Adsay therefore argued that distant metastasis might indeed represent a metachronous neoplasm rather than a metastasis of SCN [10].

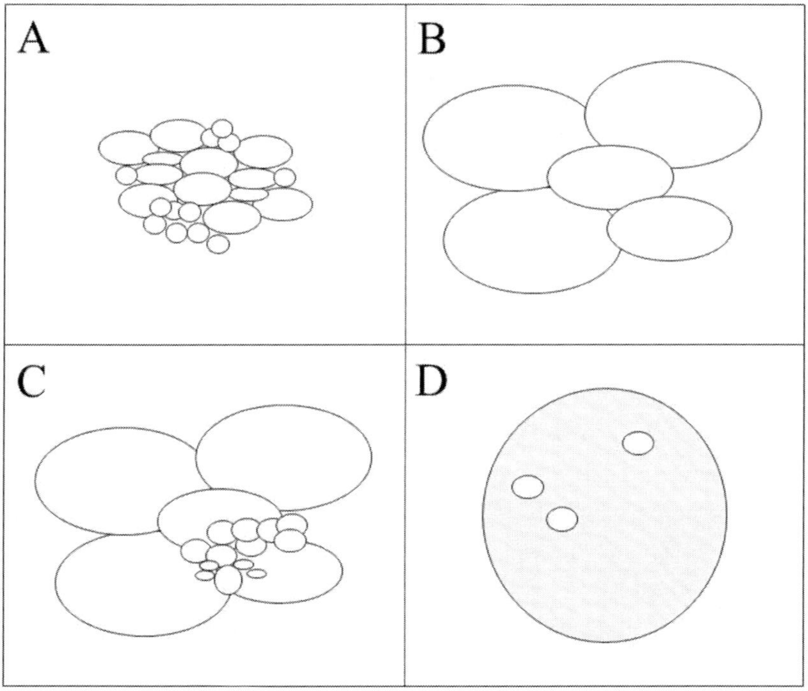

Figure 2. Four macroscopic types of SCN: microcystic (A), macrocystic (B), mixed microcystic and macrocystic (C) and solid (D) (referred to [15]).

It has to been kept in mind, that malignant SCN have nothing in common with ductal adenocarcinoma of the pancreas although ductal adenocarcinoma may appear with cystic lesions as a result of degenerative changes [17].

Contrary to the statement of Adsay the European Expert Consensus Statement on cystic tumors of the pancreas considered that SCN can show local aggressive behavior which is defined as invasion of vessels or peripancreatic lymph nodes. However, in synopsis of actual evidence, the Consensus Statement also considered that the SCN may be regarded as benign entity [5].

Clinical Characteristics of SCN

SCN are very variable in their morphology and therefore their clinical behavior. Specific laboratory values are not existent. However, present evidence gives some hint that might help in the clinical diagnosis. Review of the literature shows that SCN is a lesion that is most frequently found in women. Women are affected in 75-87% and therefore the female to male ratio is 3:1. Mean age at the time of diagnosis was 58-61 years with a very broad range from 16-99 years [6, 9, 12, 16, 18].

SCA is generally asymptomatic in around 60% of patients and is mostly discovered incidentally during imaging studies performed for symptoms not related to the pancreas [6, 9]. There was a two-fold increase in incidentally diagnosed cystic neoplasms during the last 30 years and currently, nearly 50% of resected cystic neoplasms are diagnosed this way (14). If symptoms occur these are mostly unspecific like abdominal pain that was reported in 27-71% of the patients, weight loss in 4-22%, and discomfort, nausea and vomiting in 10% [6, 9, 18]. Relatively specific symptoms are an abdominal mass (22%), obstructive jaundice (6-9%), acute pancreatitis (2-9%) and upper GI obstruction [6, 9, 18]. The mean diameter of the SCN ranges from 3.1-4.9cm [6, 9, 16]. A significant correlation between cyst size and clinical symptoms was reported [6].

Diagnosis of SCN

The European Expert Consensus Statement on SCN recommend a CT and/or an MRI scan as gold standard in the diagnosis of SCN. The experts do not see a difference between CT and MRI concerning specifity and sensitivity [5].

Previous studies showed that CT and MRI are the most frequently used imaging modalities. Jais et al. reported that preoperative evaluation included CT, MRI and EUS in 13%, CT and MRI in 17%, CT and EUS in 15%, MRI and EUS in 2%, CT alone in 47%, MRI alone in 5% and EUS alone in 1% [6]. Le Borgne et al. reported that ultrasound and CT were performed in 91%, ultrasound, CT and EUS in 28%, ERCP in 20% and MRI in 14% [9].

A CT-scan typically demonstrates a multicystic, lobulated mass within the pancreas, sometimes described as a 'bunch of grapes'. The individual cysts are typically less than 2 mm in size and greater than six in number-except for the oligocystic variety. As mentioned above, some SCN display a characteristic enhancing central scar which can show associated stellate calcification [19, 20]. In MRI SCN usually appear as a cluster of small cysts within the pancreas. There is no visible communication between the cysts and the pancreatic duct. The signal characteristics include a typically low signal in T1. The fibrous septa between the cysts may enhance on delayed contrast enhanced images using Gadolinium. In T2 the central fibrous scar has a low signal while cystic components themselves display high signal [19, 20].

When CT or MRI can not proof the diagnosis there are additional diagnostic tools that might help. Endo-ultrasound (EUS) is one of these. EUS is an invasive procedure, however, complication rate is low. Jais et al. suggested criteria for diagnosis of SCN by means of EUS. These are the existence of microcysts (2 mm or less) which are separated by thin septa, which sometimes appear as layered and a thin cyst outline wall. If these cysts are absent, a low CEA level in the cyst fluid might be considered specific for SCN [6]. The sensitivity and specifity of EUS was reported to be 56-71% and 43-97% respectively [5]. EUS is more frequently used in lesions that merit resection, and this is mirrored in the fact that most of the patients had CT or MRI prior to this modality. Fine needle aspiration (FNA) is an additional diagnostic procedure that can be helpful in diagnosis of SCN [5]. A study from Brugge et al. showed that aspiration under EUS guidance showed low mean centrations of CEA as a cyst fluid tumor marker compared to mucinous cysts [13]. Although cytological analysis can also be performed by means of FNA, cytologic analysis is acellular in 50% of cases. Because of this cytological analysis is not helpful in distinguishing SCA from mucinous cystic tumors [9].

Prognosis and Treatment of SCN

The European Experts clearly state that SCN should be considered as a benign disease and must not be resected. The presence of symptoms and the inability to exclude malignancy, however, are indications for surgery [5]. Due to the nature of the lesions, pancreas and spleen preserving procedures must be considered. In the case of malignancy suspicion, an oncological approach must be used. Recently, a decrease in operative therapy from 94% between 1990 and 1995 to 54% between 2010 and 2014 was reported [6]. Retrospective studies showed that the percentage of patients with SCN among patients with cystic tumors ranges from 10-16% in sizable surgical cohorts [5, 16]. Postoperative mortality rates after pancreatic resection for SCN were 0.5- 2.2% [6, 9, 16]. Although long-term follow-up showed no death due to SCN, the recurrence of SCA was observed in two cases [9]. Disease specific mortality was 0.1% in one study, however, this was due to a diagnostic procedure (ERCP) [6].

An actual recommendation for surgically fit patients with SCN is a follow-up program after 3-6 months if no resection is performed. The further follow-up is dependent on the growth rate of the lesion [5].

In serous cystadenocarcinomas, normal tumor follow-up should be performed. The prognosis seems to be good with the survival of patients up to nine years after resection [6]. However, data is too limited to make general statements. There is no general statement on adjuvant or neoadjuvant therapy. Adjuvant therapy can be performed in serous cystadenocarcinoma [5].

REFERENCES

[1] Distler, M; Aust, D; Weitz, J; Pilarsky, C; Grutzmann, R. Precursor lesions for sporadic pancreatic cancer: PanIN, IPMN, and MCN. *Biomed Res Int*, (2014), 474905.

[2] Grutzmann, R; Post, S; Saeger, HD; Niedergethmann, M. Intraductal papillary mucinous neoplasia (IPMN) of the pancreas: its diagnosis, treatment, and prognosis. *Dtsch Arztebl Int*, (108), 788-794.

[3] Compagno, J; Oertel, JE. Microcystic adenomas of the pancreas (glycogen-rich cystadenomas): a clinicopathologic study of 34 cases. 1978, *Am J Clin Pathol*, (69), 289-298.

[4] Morana, G; Guarise, A. Cystic tumors of the pancreas. 2006, *Cancer Imaging*, (6), 60-71.

[5] Del Chiaro, M; Verbeke, C; Salvia, R; Kloppel, G; Werner, J; McKay, C; Friess, H; Manfredi, R; Van Cutsem, E; Lohr, M; Segersvard, R. European experts consensus statement on cystic tumours of the pancreas. *Digestive and liver disease: official journal of the Italian Society of Gastroenterology and the Italian Association for the Study of the Liver*, (45), 703-711.

[6] Jais, B; Rebours, V; Malleo, G; Salvia, R; Fontana, M; Maggino, L; Bassi, C; Manfredi, R; Moran, R; Lennon, AM; Zaheer, A; Wolfgang, C; Hruban, R; Marchegiani, G; Fernandez Del Castillo, C; Brugge, W; Ha, Y; Kim, MH; Oh, D; Hirai, I; Kimura, W; Jang, JY; Kim, SW; Jung, W; Kang, H; Song, SY; Kang, CM; Lee, WJ; Crippa, S; Falconi, M; Gomatos, I; Neoptolemos, J; Milanetto, AC; Sperti, C; Ricci, C; Casadei, R; Bissolati, M; Balzano, G; Frigerio, I; Girelli, R; Delhaye, M; Bernier, B; Wang, H; Jang, KT; Song, DH; Huggett, MT; Oppong, KW; Pererva, L; Kopchak, KV; Del Chiaro, M; Segersvard, R; Lee, LS; Conwell, D; Osvaldt, A; Campos, V; Aguero Garcete, G; Napoleon, B; Matsumoto, I; Shinzeki, M;

Bolado, F; Fernandez, JM; Keane, MG; Pereira, SP; Acuna, IA; Vaquero, EC; Angiolini, MR; Zerbi, A; Tang, J; Leong, RW; Faccinetto, A; Morana, G; Petrone, MC; Arcidiacono, PG; Moon, JH; Choi, HJ; Gill, RS; Pavey, D; Ouaissi, M; Sastre, B; Spandre, M; De Angelis, CG; Rios-Vives, MA; Concepcion-Martin, M; Ikeura, T; Okazaki, K; Frulloni, L; Messina, O; Levy, P. Serous cystic neoplasm of the pancreas: a multinational study of 2622 patients under the auspices of the International Association of Pancreatology and European Pancreatic Club (European Study Group on Cystic Tumors of the Pancreas). 2015, *Gut*, (65), 305-312.

[7] Klöppel, G; Solcia, E; Longnecker, DS; Capella, C; Sobin, L. eds. *Histological Typing of Tumours of the Exocrine Pancreas*. Springer, 1996.

[8] Kosmahl, M; Pauser, U; Peters, K; Sipos, B; Luttges, J; Kremer, B; Kloppel, G. Cystic neoplasms of the pancreas and tumor-like lesions with cystic features: a review of 418 cases and a classification proposal. 2004, *Virchows Arch*, (445), 168-178.

[9] Le Borgne, J; de Calan, L; Partensky, C. Cystadenomas and cystadenocarcinomas of the pancreas: a multiinstitutional retrospective study of 398 cases. French Surgical Association. 1999, *Ann Surg*, (230), 152-161.

[10] Volkan Adsay, N. Cystic lesions of the pancreas. 2007, *Mod Pathol*, (20 Suppl 1), S71-93.

[11] Kosmahl, M; Wagner, J; Peters, K; Sipos, B; Kloppel, G. Serous cystic neoplasms of the pancreas: an immunohistochemical analysis revealing alpha-inhibin, neuron-specific enolase, and MUC6 as new markers. 2004, *Am J Surg Pathol*, (28), 339-346.

[12] Basturk, O; Coban, I; Adsay, NV. Pancreatic cysts: pathologic classification, differential diagnosis, and clinical implications. 2009, *Archives of pathology & laboratory medicine*, (133), 423-438.

[13] Brugge, WR; Lewandrowski, K; Lee-Lewandrowski, E; Centeno, BA; Szydlo, T; Regan, S; del Castillo, CF; Warshaw, AL. Diagnosis of pancreatic cystic neoplasms: a report of the cooperative pancreatic cyst study. 2004, *Gastroenterology*, (126), 1330-1336.

[14] Mohr, VH; Vortmeyer, AO; Zhuang, Z; Libutti, SK; Walther, MM; Choyke, PL; Zbar, B; Linehan, WM; Lubensky, IA. Histopathology and molecular genetics of multiple cysts and microcystic (serous) adenomas of the pancreas in von Hippel-Lindau patients. 2000, *Am J Pathol*, (157), 1615-1621.

[15] Kimura, W; Moriya, T; Hirai, I; Hanada, K; Abe, H; Yanagisawa, A; Fukushima, N; Ohike, N; Shimizu, M; Hatori, T; Fujita, N; Maguchi, H; Shimizu, Y; Yamao, K; Sasaki, T; Naito, Y; Tanno, S; Tobita, K; Tanaka, M. Multicenter study of serous cystic neoplasm of the Japan pancreas society. *Pancreas*, (41), 380-387.

[16] Valsangkar, NP; Morales-Oyarvide, V; Thayer, SP; Ferrone, CR; Wargo, JA; Warshaw, AL. Fernandez-del Castillo C, 851 resected cystic tumors of the pancreas: a 33-year experience at the Massachusetts General Hospital. *Surgery*, (152), S4-12.

[17] Adsay, NV; Klimstra, DS. Cystic forms of typically solid pancreatic tumors. 2000, *Semin Diagn Pathol*, (17), 81-88.

[18] Galanis, C; Zamani, A; Cameron, JL; Campbell, KA; Lillemoe, KD; Caparrelli, D; Chang, D; Hruban, RH; Yeo, CJ. Resected serous cystic neoplasms of the pancreas: a review of 158 patients with recommendations for treatment. 2007, *J Gastrointest Surg*, (11), 820-826.

[19] Choi, JY; Kim, MJ; Lee, JY; Lim, JS; Chung, JJ; Kim, KW; Yoo, HS. Typical and atypical manifestations of serous cystadenoma of the pancreas: imaging findings with pathologic correlation. 2009, *AJR Am J Roentgenol*, (193), 136-142.

[20] Kim, HJ; Lee, DH; Ko, YT; Lim, JW; Kim, HC; Kim, KW. CT of serous cystadenoma of the pancreas and mimicking masses. 2008, *AJR Am J Roentgenol*, (190), 406-412.

In: Cystic Tumors of the Pancreas
Editor: Robert Grützmann
ISBN: 978-1-53612-523-8

Chapter 9

INTRADUCTAL PAPILLARY MUCINOUS NEOPLASIA (IPMN)

Georg Ferdinand Weber**, MD, PhD and Robert Grützmann, MD, PhD, MBA
Department of Surgery, Friedrich-Alexander University of Erlangen-Nuremberg, Erlangen, Germany

ABSTRACT

The diagnosis of intraductal mucinous neoplasia (IPMN) is increasing. Here, we summarize existing data on the definition, detection and treatment of main duct-IPMNs (MD-IPMN) and branch duct-IPMNs (BD-IPMN). Because of the risk for malignant transformation, the Sendai criteria has been established, including guidelines for the treatment of the various IPMNs. However, recent evidence is challenging the accuracy of this critera, especially in predicting the risk for malignant transformation in Sendai positive and negative BD-IPMNs.

Keywords: MD-IPMN, BD-IPMN, Sendai criteria, high risk stigmata, worrisome feature, diagnostic accuracy, treatment algorhythm

* Corresponding Author Email: georg.weber@uk-erlangen.de.

INTRODUCTION

The diagnosis of intraductal papillary mucinous neoplasia (IPMN) has been dramatically increasing in the past few decades [1]. This is not due to an actual increase of the prevalence itself but most likely due to technical advances in the diagnostic of even small pancreatic IPMNs and a better awareness of this disease in the community [2–4]. Histopathological and genetic analyses of resected tumor specimens have led to a better understanding of the mechanisms for malignant transformation of IPMNs [5–11]. In addition, risk stratification guidelines for IPMNs are evolving, affecting directly the treatment strategies [12, 13]. Within this chapter, we will give a comprehensive overview about new findings regarding the diagnosis and treatment of IPMNs.

The International Consensus Guidelines of 2012 for the management of IPMNs and MCN of the pancreas include recommendations for the classification, diagnosis, treatment and follow-up procedures for IPMNs [13]. However, the guidelines are designated still as a 'consensus', rather than 'evidence-based'. Distinct subtypes of IPMNs include main duct-IPMNs (MD-IPMNs), branch duct-IPMNs (BD-IPMNs), and mixed type-IPMNs (MT-IPMNs) [14]. Typically, patients with MD-IPMNs show symptoms like epigastric pain, weight loss, jaundice, diabetes or pancreatitis with decreasing frequency for patients with MT- and BD-IPMNs. MD-IPMNs have been described to be one of three precursor lesions of pancreatic adenocarcinoma besides PanIN and Mucinous Cystic Neoplasm (MCN) because of their capacity for malignant transformation, which is much higher as compared to BD- and MT-IPMNs [15, 16]. As all three IPMN types have the capacity for malignant transformation, an early detection of these lesions followed by an accurate risk stratification and therapy regimen is of utmost importance. However, the distinction of MD-IPMNs, BD-IPMNs, and MT-IPMNs can be difficult [16]. In the following sections, we discuss the two main types of IPMNs regarding definition, detection, treatment, and follow-up strategies.

Main Duct-IPMN (MD-IPMN)

Definition

MD-IPMNs are defined as a segmental or diffuse dilation of the main pancreatic duct (MPD) >5mm without other causes of obstruction. An MPD dilation of 5-9mm is considered as a 'worrisome feature', a MPD diameter of ≥10mm is considered as a 'high-risk stigmata' [13]. The following table will give a comprehensive overview of additional 'worrisome features' and 'high risk stigmata'.

Table 1. The Sendai criteria: 'high risk stigmata' and 'worrisome feature' [13]

high-risk stigmata	worrisome feature
enhancing solid components	cyst ≥3cm
main pancreatic duct ≥10mm	thickened and enhancing cyst wall
obstructive jaundice	non-enhancing mural nodules
	main pancreatic duct 5-9mm
	abrupt change in the main pancreatic duct caliber with distal pancreatic atrophy
	lymphadenopathy

Detection

MD-IPMNs can be detected by CT, MRI and MRCP. The MRCP is very useful to distinguish especially between MD-IPMNs from BD-IPMNs. Due to high malignant transformation of MD-IPMNs the precise differentiation of MD-IPMNs and BD-IPMNs is crucial. Thereby, the dilation of the MPD is the most important factor for risk stratification and decision making. In addition, by using MRI enhanced solid components of the cyst can be detected that are considered to be 'high-risk stigmata' [13].

Clinically, patients with MD-IPMNs present with abdominal pain (55%), weight loss (45%), jaundice (17%) and acute pancreatitis (15%) [17–19]. Primarily, MD-IPMNs are located in the pancreatic head. In approximately 8% the entire pancreas is affected. Endoscopically, an altered major duodenal papilla can be detected in around 30% of all MD-IPMNs with increasing numbers up to 75% when an invasive IPMN is existent [20]. Table 2 gives a comprehensive overview of diagnostic algorithms to identify IPMNs.

Table 2. Diagnostic algorithm. Adapted from Grützmann et al. [21]

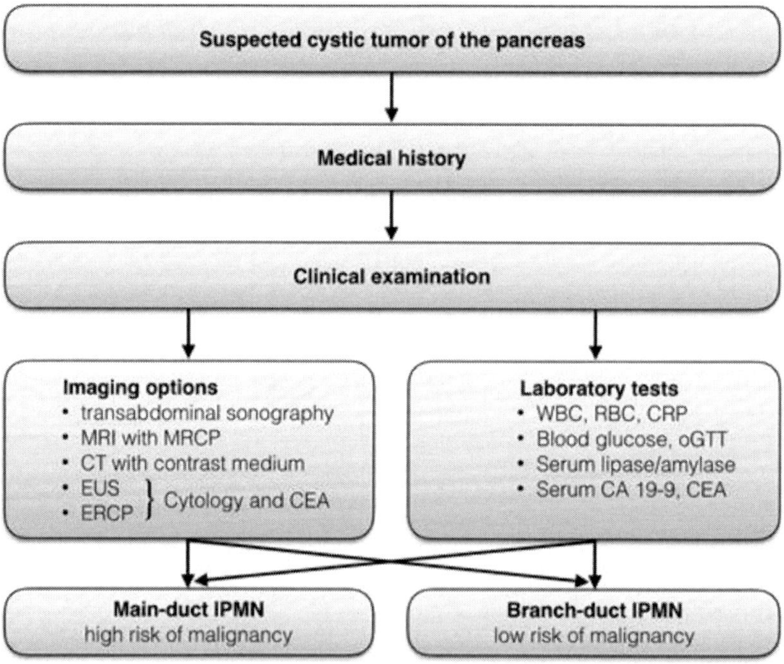

Treatment

The malignant transformation of MD-IPMNs into high grade dysplasia and invasive adenocarcinomas has been detected in 62% of all resected

MD-IPMNs [13]. In addition, the precise preoperative diagnosis of an invasive adenocarcinoma within an existing MD-IPMN is still difficult [22]. Therefore, an oncologic resection is recommended for all MD-IPMNs in patients with justifiable preoperative risk [13] (Table 3).

The surgical therapy of MD-IPMNs is dependent on the location of MD-IPMNs and their suspicion for malignancy. For MD-IPMNs located in the pancreatic head a pylorus preserving partial pancreato-duodenectomy (70%), for MD-IPMNs located in the pancreatic tail a left pancreatic resection with splenectomy (25%) is recommended [13]. The main goal for the surgical treatment is achieving a negative resection margin. This requires to perform frozen section examination of the resection margin intra-operatively to ultimately decide for the resection line. In the case of a positive resection margin with detection of high-grade dysplasia, an additional resection (normally a slice of 2cm) should be performed until a negative or at least moderate-grade dysplasia resection margin is confirmed [7, 13]. But what is the correct treatment when still low-, moderate-, or even high-grade dysplasia is detected in the resection margin after performed re-resection. The results discussing the different options are still controversial [13]. The decision to extend the resection, in rare cases ultimately to a total pancreatectomy, has to be made individually. So far, the consensus guidelines suggests that a total pancreatectomy in selected younger patients can be considered even in cases of low- or moderate-grade dysplasia due to their probably better handling of the complexity of brittle diabetes and exocrine insufficiency [13]. At which dysplasia grade a pancreatectomy has to be considered in older patients still need to be evaluated in more detail. Other surgical procedures include duodenum-preserving resections or segmental resections. However, if a positive resection margin is detected the extension of the resection line will be more complicated, therefore, these surgical procedures should be performed only in an individual approach. As for preoperative undetected malignant transformation, a lymphadenectomy should be performed regularly as of the risk [13, 16, 21].

Table 3. Therapeutic algorithm. Adapted from Grützmann et al. [21]

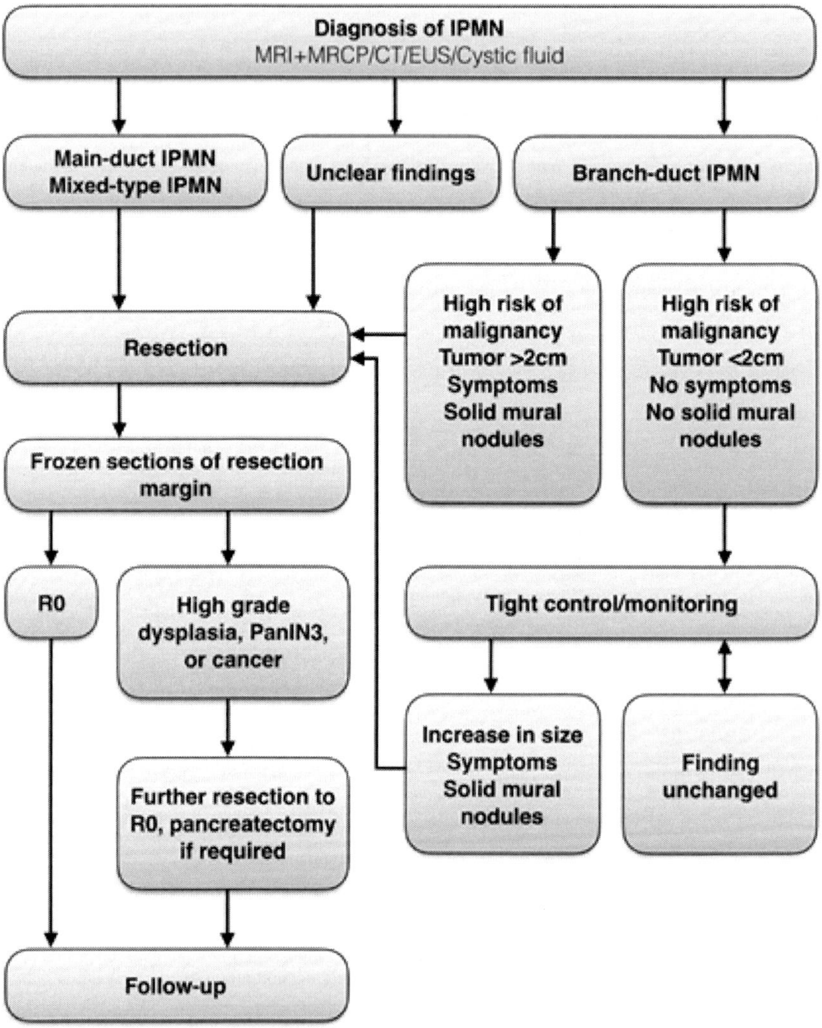

Smaller MD-IPMNs are more difficult to classify [22]. The heterogeneity of small IPMNs regarding to their capacity to evolve into an invasive carcinoma is making it necessary to develop an accurate risk stratification system. In addition, if ‘worrisome’ features are not detectable in small MD-IPMNs decision making regarding to a wait-and-see concept with regular follow-up appointments or surgical resection gets even more tricky. The easiest solution, of course, would be to perform surgery in all cases of MD-IPMNs. Even small MD-IPMNs with a main pancreatic duct between 5-9mm of size have been shown to bear a significant risk for malignant transformation [23]. However, the frequency of malignant transformation within small MD-IPMNs is only up to 25% leading to an over treatment for 75% of patients in those cases. We have to keep in mind that surgery is followed by various morbidities and a low, but still indisputable, mortality rate [24]. From an ethical point of view it is important to understand what this means for all patients with MD-IPMNs that have been resected, however, their post-surgical histopathological feature shows a small to very low probability for malignant transformation or even have been mis-diagnosed preoperatively [22]. The other side of the coin would be initiating a wait-and-see concept, even for small MD-IPMNs that cannot be stratified correctly with the actual 'worrisome features' of the Sendai criteria. This would mean that patients with 'ticking time bombs' will get included into wait-and-see concepts risking the development of invasive adenocarcinoma and hence, reduced survival[25]. Although regular follow-up is recommended, the correct time point for resection can be missed. We learn that both approaches are not perfect, however, most pancreatic surgeons agree to perform surgery in case of uncertainty in otherwise fit patients until better risk stratification concepts are available [16, 21].

BRANCH DUCT-IPMN (BD-IPMN)

Definition

Pancreatic cysts of >5mm in diameter with communication to the MPD should be considered as BD-IPMNs [13].

Detection

The gold standard for the detection of BD-IPMNs is the MRCP [13, 14]. The typical morphology, the connection duct to the MPD without dilation, and sometimes the location in multiple sites can be most accurately detected by MRCP. In addition, by using MRI and EUS the quality and size of the cyst can be identified more easily [20]. However, the uncertainty in the differentiation of MD-IPMNs from BD-IPMNs and if BD-IPMNs show signs of malignancy - even after the use of all possible diagnostic procedures - leads to a diagnostic accuracy for BD-IPMNs of only 60-80% [22, 26–28].

For a better risk stratification of IPMNs the Sendai criteria has been established in 2006 and updated in 2012 [12, 13]. Within the consensus guidelines 'worrisome features' and 'high-risk stigmata' have been developed (Table 1). The mentioned criteria can be identified using CT, MRI, and MRCP. In cases of BD-IPMNs with positive 'worrisome features' an additional EUS should be performed [20]. Thereby, a thickened enhanced cyst wall, non-enhanced mural nodules, or a suspicious cytology can be detected, all of which are 'worrisome features'. In addition, the analysis of CEA and amylase levels in the cystic fluid can help to differentiate various cystic lesions in the pancreas. Several studies have shown that the CEA levels correlate with the risk for malignant transformation [21]. High CEA levels within the cystic fluid should therefore be considered as a premalignant transformation and a surgical resection should be performed [13]. For an even better risk stratification of cystic lesions of the pancreas the molecular analysis of cystic fluids might play an important role in the future [5, 8]. To better predict the risk for malignancy in patients with BD-IPMN a recently constructed nomogram might be of help [29].

The existence of risk factors in BD-IPMNs is most important for the correct treatment as those risk factors can partially predict the likelihood for malignant transformation leading to a more aggressive treatment strategy. In addition, in 20-40% of all BD-IPMNs more than 2 BD-IPMNs can be detected in multiple locations. This, compared to the uni-localised

MCN, might be depended on a 'field defect' of the entire epithelium of the pancreatic duct system having impact on the follow-up regimen. Patients with resected non-invasive BD-IPMNs should therefore be assigned to regular follow-ups to detect possible new BD-IPMNs in the future [13].

Treatment

The Sendai criteria allows the most precise analysis of BD-IPMNs. Following this criteria, BD-IPMNs with 'high-risk stigmata' should be resected immediately without any further diagnostics in consideration of the patient's own risk factors (Table 3). In cases of BD-IPMNs with positive 'worrisome features' a surgical resection should be recommended considering the age of the patient, the location, size and growth dynamic of the cyst, and further co-morbidities of the patient. Therefore, the decisions for surgical treatment for BD-IPMNs with 'worrisome features' is always made individually. If none of those criterias are present, the patient should be appointed to a follow-up regimen dependent on the size of the cyst and age of the patient [13]. However, recent data challenge the actual consensus guidelines because of lacking adequate sensitivity and specificity [28, 30]. Another questions is the treatment regarding to single and multiple lesions in the pancreas.

a) Single lesion: several requirements exist for the resection of a single lesion. First, achieving an R0 resection is of utmost importance and has to be the highest rated goal. Second, the procedure with the lowest complications has to be chosen to achieve R0 resection. Third, preservation of pancreatic tissue has to be considered in the initial planning of the surgical procedure [31].
b) Multiple lesions: if multiple lesion are detected every lesion has to be evaluated regarding to the existing risk factors. In case of high risk for malignancy for one of the detected lesions the possibility of a surgical procedure should be discussed with the patient.

Thereby, the other lesions need to be evaluated regarding to their proximity to the lesion with the highest risk for malignancy. In case of close proximity an extended surgical approach might achieve the resection of all lesions without performing an pancreatectomy. If the other detected lesion/s are in distance to the lesion with high risk for malignancy the enucleation of those lesions can be discussed to preserve pancreatic tissue and prevent the necessity for a total pancreatectomy [31]. In case of two or more lesions with high risk for malignancy a total pancreatectomy should be performed [13, 31]. In case non of the lesions have signs for malignancy a watch and wait concept can be discussed, however, the risk for malignant transformation has still to be taken into account [28].

Discussion

Although the Sendai criteria have increased the awareness of cystic lesions and their treatment dependent on the risk stratification, several questions remain. As we have learned, MD-IPMNs as well as BD-IPMNs with 'high-risk stigmata' should be directly treated by surgical resection. In addition, MD-IPMNs and BD-IPMNs with 'worrisome features', dependent on the patient's age, co-morbidities, and clinical appearance, will as well benefit from a surgical resection due to their possible malignant transformation. However, there are still ongoing discussions regarding the treatment of various MD- and BD-IPMNs dependent on patient's age and co-morbidities.

It is still unclear at which exact dilation of the MPD in MD-IPMNs a surgical resection should be performed. Although 'worrisome features' and 'high-risk stigmata' have been established with recommendations for treatment strategies, it is still an individual decision regarding exact dilation of the MPD and the location of the MD-IPMN. As an example, is a surgical approach due to a MD-IPMN in the pancreatic head with a dilation of 8mm in an 85 year old patient with minor co-morbidities and no symptoms the ideal treatment? For the optimal decision, several pieces of information are necessary: The life expectancy of the patient, the exact risk for malignant transformation of the MD-IPMN, the growth dynamic of the MD-IPMN, the post-surgical morbidity and quality-of-life, and the expected mortality rate (within the designated centre). Only some of this information will be available, hence it will always be an imperfect decision for every patient. We have to learn more about the biology of the disease, the various histological variances as well as the genetic drivers for malignant transformation to get closer to an ideal treatment concept.

The differentiation of BD-IPMNs from MD-IPMNs is of the utmost clinical relevance, as BD-IPMNs have a significantly lower malignant transformation rate compared to MD-IPMNs (20-25% vs. 60-75%, respectively) [13, 18, 23, 28, 32]; however, the treatment strategy for BD-IPMNs are still controversially discussed. In a recent meta-analysis the risk of pancreatic malignancy and mortality in BD-IPMNs undergoing surveillance has been assessed. The authors concluded that the non-operative management of low-risk (Sendai negative) BD-IPMNs is safe [33]. But evidence exists that even Sendai-negative BD-IPMNs have the capacity for malignant transformation developing into a malignant disease.

Although it is recommended that patients with Sendai negative BD-IPMNs should receive regular follow-up diagnostics, the risk factors included in the Sendai criteria still lack specificity and sensitivity and are not always accurate enough, especially for smaller lesions [13, 28, 34]. Recent evidence shows BD-IPMN associated carcinomas from Sendai negative BD-IPMNs is rare, but higher than it was estimated [28, 35]. It has to be discussed if young patients with Sendai negative BD-IPMNs should be recommended for a surgical prophylactic resection due to their long life expectancy, and therefore whether or not they are at risk for malignant transformation [36]. Although the risk for malignant transformation has been shown to be small, the event of a missed malignant transformation will possibly lower the life expectancy of these patients dramatically. However, this is just one side of the coin. The justification for surgical treatment of BD-IPMNs showing no risk parameters in young patients is the expected malignant transformation at some point. However, as we do not understand the timeline of malignant transformation of these Sendai negative BD-IPMNs yet, over-treatment of many patients will occur as some of them probably would never have developed a malignant disease, and many patients will have been misdiagnosed [22]. It has to be considered that patients undergoing surgery show as well postoperative morbidity, which alters the quality-of-life. The younger the patient, the bigger the effect will be if postoperative morbidity occurs. Finally, the mortality rate of pancreatic surgery in a non-malignant state is low, but not zero. This means that patients will die due to over-treatment because of the fear of developing a malignant disease at some point in their lives. It has been shown that surveillance of BD-IPMNs leads to a risk for developing a malignant disease in 1.4% during 5 years [37]. However, this is comparable to the 90-day mortality rate for pancreatic surgery in high-volume hospitals. Therefore, from our point of view, a prophylactic resection of Sendai negative BD-IPMNs cannot be recommended at this moment.

REFERENCES

[1] Kimura W, Nagai H, Kuroda A, Muto T, Esaki Y. Analysis of small cystic lesions of the pancreas. *Int J Pancreatol.* 1995;18:197-206.

[2] Sohn TA, Yeo CJ, Cameron JL et al. Intraductal papillary mucinous neoplasms of the pancreas: an updated experience. *Ann Surg.* 2004;239:788-97; discussion 797.

[3] Laffan TA, Horton KM, Klein AP et al. Prevalence of unsuspected pancreatic cysts on MDCT. *AJR Am J Roentgenol.* 2008;191:802-807.

[4] Farrell JJ. Prevalence, Diagnosis and Management of Pancreatic Cystic Neoplasms: Current Status and Future Directions. *Gut Liver.* 2015;9:571-589.

[5] Wu J, Matthaei H, Maitra A et al. Recurrent GNAS mutations define an unexpected pathway for pancreatic cyst development. *Sci Transl Med.* 2011;3:92ra66.

[6] Distler M, Kersting S, Niedergethmann M et al. Pathohistological subtype predicts survival in patients with intraductal papillary mucinous neoplasm (IPMN) of the pancreas. *Ann Surg.* 2013;258:324-330.

[7] Distler M, Welsch T, Aust D, Weitz J, Grutzmann R. [Intraductal papillary mucinous neoplasm of the pancreas (IPMN)--standards and new aspects]. *Zentralbl Chir.* 2014;139:308-317.

[8] Yu J, Sadakari Y, Shindo K et al. Digital next-generation sequencing identifies low-abundance mutations in pancreatic juice samples collected from the duodenum of patients with pancreatic cancer and intraductal papillary mucinous neoplasms. *Gut.* 2016.

[9] Mino-Kenudson M, Fernandez-del Castillo C, Baba Y et al. Prognosis of invasive intraductal papillary mucinous neoplasm depends on histological and precursor epithelial subtypes. *Gut.* 2011;60:1712-1720.

[10] Adsay NV, Merati K, Basturk O et al. Pathologically and biologically distinct types of epithelium in intraductal papillary mucinous neoplasms: delineation of an "intestinal" pathway of carcinogenesis in the pancreas. *Am J Surg Pathol.* 2004;28:839-848.

[11] Nissim S, Idos GE, Wu B. Genetic markers of malignant transformation in intraductal papillary mucinous neoplasm of the pancreas: a meta-analysis. *Pancreas.* 2012;41:1195-1205.

[12] Tanaka M, Chari S, Adsay V et al. International consensus guidelines for management of intraductal papillary mucinous neoplasms and mucinous cystic neoplasms of the pancreas. *Pancreatology.* 2006;6:17-32.

[13] Tanaka M, Fernandez-del Castillo C, Adsay V et al. International consensus guidelines 2012 for the management of IPMN and MCN of the pancreas. *Pancreatology.* 2012;12:183-197.

[14] Kim KW, Park SH, Pyo J et al. Imaging features to distinguish malignant and benign branch-duct type intraductal papillary mucinous neoplasms of the pancreas: a meta-analysis. *Ann Surg.* 2014;259:72-81.

[15] Nagai K, Doi R, Kida A et al. Intraductal papillary mucinous neoplasms of the pancreas: clinicopathologic characteristics and long-term follow-up after resection. *World J Surg.* 2008;32:271-8; discussion 279.

[16] Grutzmann R, Niedergethmann M, Pilarsky C, Kloppel G, Saeger HD. Intraductal papillary mucinous tumors of the pancreas: biology, diagnosis, and treatment. *Oncologist.* 2010;15:1294-1309.

[17] Kosmahl M, Pauser U, Anlauf M et al. [Cystic pancreas tumors and their classification: features old and new]. *Pathologe.* 2005;26:22-30.

[18] Salvia R, Fernandez-del Castillo C, Bassi C et al. Main-duct intraductal papillary mucinous neoplasms of the pancreas: clinical predictors of malignancy and long-term survival following resection. *Ann Surg.* 2004;239:678-85; discussion 685.

[19] Crippa S, Fernandez-Del Castillo C, Salvia R et al. Mucin-producing neoplasms of the pancreas: an analysis of distinguishing clinical and epidemiologic characteristics. *Clin Gastroenterol Hepatol.* 2010;8:213-219.

[20] Tanaka M. Current roles of endoscopy in the management of intraductal papillary mucinous neoplasm of the pancreas. *Dig Endosc.* 2015;27:450-457.

[21] Grutzmann R, Post S, Saeger HD, Niedergethmann M. Intraductal papillary mucinous neoplasia (IPMN) of the pancreas: its diagnosis, treatment, and prognosis. *Dtsch Arztebl Int.* 2011;108:788-794.

[22] Del Chiaro M, Segersvard R, Pozzi Mucelli R et al. Comparison of preoperative conference-based diagnosis with histology of cystic tumors of the pancreas. *Ann Surg Oncol.* 2014;21:1539-1544.

[23] Hackert T, Fritz S, Klauss M et al. Main-duct Intraductal Papillary Mucinous Neoplasm: High Cancer Risk in Duct Diameter of 5 to 9 mm. *Ann Surg.* 2015;262:875-80; discussion 880.

[24] Nimptsch U, Krautz C, Weber GF, Mansky T, Grutzmann R. Nationwide In-hospital Mortality Following Pancreatic Surgery in Germany is Higher than Anticipated. *Ann Surg.* 2016;264:1082-1090.

[25] Del Chiaro M, Ateeb Z, Hansson MR et al. Survival Analysis and Risk for Progression of Intraductal Papillary Mucinous Neoplasia of

the Pancreas (IPMN) Under Surveillance: A Single-Institution Experience. *Ann Surg Oncol*. 2017;24:1120-1126.

[26] Fernandez-del Castillo C, Adsay NV. Intraductal papillary mucinous neoplasms of the pancreas. *Gastroenterology*. 2010;139:708-13, 713.e1.

[27] Kawada N, Uehara H, Nagata S, Tsuchishima M, Tsutsumi M, Tomita Y. Predictors of malignancy in branch duct intraductal papillary mucinous neoplasm of the pancreas. *JOP*. 2014;15:459-464.

[28] Heckler M, Michalski CW, Schaefle S, Kaiser J, Buchler MW, Hackert T. The Sendai and Fukuoka consensus criteria for the management of branch duct IPMN - A meta-analysis on their accuracy. *Pancreatology*. 2017;17:255-262.

[29] Jang JY, Park T, Lee S et al. Proposed Nomogram Predicting the Individual Risk of Malignancy in the Patients With Branch Duct Type Intraductal Papillary Mucinous Neoplasms of the Pancreas. *Ann Surg*. 2016.

[30] Kobayashi G, Fujita N, Maguchi H et al. Natural history of branch duct intraductal papillary mucinous neoplasm with mural nodules: a Japan Pancreas Society multicenter study. *Pancreas*. 2014;43:532-538.

[31] Turrini O, Schmidt CM, Pitt HA et al. Side-branch intraductal papillary mucinous neoplasms of the pancreatic head/uncinate: resection or enucleation. *HPB* (Oxford). 2011;13:126-131.

[32] Rodriguez JR, Salvia R, Crippa S et al. Branch-duct intraductal papillary mucinous neoplasms: observations in 145 patients who underwent resection. *Gastroenterology*. 2007;133:72-9; quiz 309.

[33] Crippa S, Capurso G, Camma C, Delle Fave G, Castillo CF, Falconi M. Risk of pancreatic malignancy and mortality in branch-duct IPMNs undergoing surveillance: A systematic review and meta-analysis. *Dig Liver Dis*. 2016;48:473-479.

[34] Tanaka M. Controversies in the management of pancreatic IPMN. *Nat Rev Gastroenterol Hepatol*. 2011;8:56-60.

[35] Cauley CE, Waters JA, Dumas RP et al. Outcomes of primary surveillance for intraductal papillary mucinous neoplasm. *J Gastrointest Surg.* 2012;16:258-67; discussion 266.

[36] Lee T, Kim HJ, Park SK et al. Natural courses of branch duct intraductal papillary mucinous neoplasm. *Langenbecks Arch Surg.* 2017.

[37] Malleo G, Marchegiani G, Borin A et al. Observational study of the incidence of pancreatic and extrapancreatic malignancies during surveillance of patients with branch-duct intraductal papillary mucinous neoplasm. *Ann Surg.* 2015;261:984-990.

In: Cystic Tumors of the Pancreas
Editor: Robert Grützmann
ISBN: 978-1-53612-523-8

Chapter 10

MUCINOUS CYSTIC NEOPLASMS

Katherine Albutt, MD, MPH and Cristina Ferrone*, MD

Department of General and Gastrointestinal Surgery
Surgical Oncology, Massachusetts General Hospital,
Boston, MA, US

ABSTRACT

Mucinous cystic neoplasms (MCNs) are the second most common mucinous pancreatic cystic neopslasm and have significant malignant potential. Typically lined by a mucin-producing ductal epithelium with an ovarian-type sroma, MCNs almost exclusively occur in women and have a peak incidence in the 5th decade. This chapter reviews the epidemiology, diagnostic work up, pathologic features, and management of MCNs in detail.

Keywords: mucinous cystic neoplasm, pancreatic cystic neoplasm, mucinous cystadenoma, mucinous cystadenocarcinoma

* Corresponding Author Email: cferrone@harvard.mgh.edu.

Introduction

Mucinous cystic neoplasms (MCNs) are cystic neoplasms lined by columnar, mucin-producing ductal epithelium with an underlying ovarian-type stroma. MCNs do not usually communicate with the pancreatic duct. They are the second most common mucinous pancreatic cystic neoplasm and have significant malignant potential.

Epidemiology

Pancreatic cystic neoplasms of all varieties are being diagnosed with increasing frequency in large part due to the availability and widespread use of axial imaging. As with other pancreatic cystic neoplasms, MCNs are most frequently detected when abdominal imaging is performed for other reasons. When symptoms are present, they are often non-specific. That being said, patients may present with abdominal pain, recurrent pancreatitis, gastric outlet obstruction, a palpable mass, jaundice, weight loss, or other ill-defined symptoms [1]. Their larger size renders them more symptomatic than some of their smaller PCN counterparts. Up to 30% of patients, however, may be asymptomatic [2]. MCNs almost exclusively occur in women (>95%) and are most common in those older than 40 years of age with a peak incidence in the 5th decade. The average age at diagnosis is 53 years [2].

Precise estimates for prevalence are not available. A retrospective case series of 850 patients suggested that 16-23% of patients undergoing surgical resection for a PCN had a mucinous cystic neoplasm (noting that this series only evaluated resected PCNs and thus likely overestimates the relative frequency of this lesion) [3]. Other estimates suggest MCNs may account for up to half of all primary PCNs [4]. Among patients evaluated for PCNs, the likelihood of the cyst being mucinous was higher for asymptomatic than symptomatic cysts, 28% versus 16% respectively [5]. It is relatively easy to distinguish MCNs from other PCNs based on their mucin-producing columnar epithelium, however they are somewhat harder to separate from pancreatic pseudocysts.

Diagnosis

If not already obtained, the first step in the diagnostic algorithm is to obtain cross-sectional imaging. Appropriate imaging modalities for PCNs include magnetic resonance imaging (MRI) with magnetic resonance cholangiopancreatography (MRCP) or a pancreatic-protocol computed tomography (CT) scan. Contrast-enhanced CT is the test of choice in MCNs given their classic appearance – a septated cystic lesion with a small number of discrete compartments (although they can be unilocular) +/- eccentric calcifications (seen in up to 15% of patients) [6, 7]. Septae are best visualized on CT after administration of intravenous contrast. On MRI, the cysts appear bright on T2 weighted images. Radiographic findings suggestive of a higher risk of malignant transformation include larger size, thick or irregular cyst wall, internal solid component or mass, calcification of the cyst wall, and evidence of local invasion [8]. Peripheral eggshell calcifications are a worrisome feature that is specific to MCNs and highly predictive of cancer [9].

After obtaining cross-sectional imaging, the optimal diagnostic approach for evaluation is a subject of ongoing debate, seeking to balance the risk of malignancy with unnecessary, and sometimes invasive, surveillance and testing. In patients where imaging does not make the diagnosis an endoscopic ultrasound with fine-needle aspiration (EUS-FNA) should be considered. FNA can confirm the presence of mucin and can often make the diagnosis of MCN. Since these lesions have significant malignant potential they should all be removed. If the diagnosis of MCN vs intraductal papillary mucinous tumor (IPMN) cannot be made then the American Gastroenterological Association 2015 guidelines should be followed. Lesions with concerning features (solid component, pancreatic ductal dilation, symptoms, family history of pancreatic malignancy) should be surgically removed [10].

High-quality ultrasonographic imaging of the pancreas and the ability to directly sample pancreatic lesions are the two principle benefits of EUS-FNA. Typical EUS findings of MCNs are thin-walled, septated viscous fluid-filled cavities. Cyst fluid can be analyzed for a variety of markers – tumor and molecular markers as well as cytology. The typical cystic fluid aspirated from MCNs is a viscous aspirate containing thick mucin or a mixture of mucin and necrotic debris. Aspirates taken from solid components within the cyst have a high yield for malignancy. Staining for mucin is positive in <50% and the CEA level is typically high (>200 ng/mL). Numerous studies have documented that MCNs are typically associated with higher levels of CEA in their cystic fluid, however the optimal cutoff level for CEA remains a subject of ongoing debate. There is some expert consensus, however, that higher levels of CEA are almost exclusively seen in mucin-producing lesions. Many practitioners, particularly in the US, use a CEA level of 192 ng/ml as a relatively sensitive (75%) and specific (84%) test for differentiating mucinous from non-mucinous cystic neoplasms with an overall diagnostic accuracy of almost 80% for mucinous lesions [11, 12]. The negative predictive value, however, is low with up to 20% of mucin-producing lesions having a normal CEA level [5]. Amylase activity is not usually elevated.

A variety of other markers including fluid DNA, glucose levels, and mucin profiling, have been used to differentiate mucinous from non-mucinous lesions with varying efficacy. Although the clinical utility of such markers remains somewhat unclear, mucinous PCNs are often associated with KRAS mutations as well as high-amplitude allelic loss of tumor suppressor genes, which was directly associated with malignant potential [13].

PATHOLOGY

According to the World Health Organization histological classification scheme for PCNs, the term mucinous cystic neoplasm includes mucinous cystadenoma, mucinous cystic neoplasm with moderate dysplasia, and mucinous cystadenocarcinoma of both invasive and non-invasive forms [14]. Historically, these neoplasms had been classified in stages – adenoma, borderline, and malignant (carcinoma in situ and invasive cancer) [15]. Available series have documented carcinoma in situ in 5% to 27% of MCNs and invasive carcinoma in 15% to 40% [15]. As described above, cyst fluid can be analyzed for cytology, tumor markers, and molecular markers. Typical MCN cytology demonstrates columnar cells with varying levels of atypia. Unfortunately, with FNA the specimen may be paucicellular, limiting the diagnostic yield. If mucin-containing cells are visualized, the cytological specimen may assist in diagnosis although the sensitivity is low. In the case of mucinous lesions, FNA portends a sensitivity and specificity of 35% and 83%, respectively for detecting MCNs [11]. Diagnostic yield may be further improved by the addition of cytology brushing for diagnosing mucinous lesions, as available evidence suggests cytobrushings were significantly more likely to detect intracellular mucin than FNA [16].

Macroscopically, MCNs present as well-encapsulated spherical masses, typically containing multiple individual cysts. Ranging up to 25cm in size, MCNs are commonly between 8 and 10cm [17]. They generally contain fewer than six individual cysts, with each individual cyst usually being >2cm. Notably, MCNs tend to arise in the pancreatic tail and body (~95%) and do not usually communicate with the pancreatic duct [8].

They have a dense mesenchymal ovarian-like stroma, a pathognomonic and requisite feature [8, 18]. Nearly all MCNs are surrounded by a thick layer of spindle cells containing receptors for progesterone and estrogen, possibly due to incorporation of ectopic ovarian stroma during embryogenesis. Malignancies arising within MCNs almost always originate within the mucinous transitional epithelium and are proliferative in nature. MCNs are classified according to the grade of dysplasia ranging from benign to MCNs with dysplasia to carcinoma in situ or invasive carcinoma. Carcinoma, noninvasive and invasive, is estimated to be present in 6-40% of MCNs, depending on classification and grouping of a true invasive adenocarcinoma [8, 18]. Often these proliferative changes coexist, and as such the tumor grade is based on the greatest atypia/dysplasia. A Mayo clinic histopathologic scheme separates MCNs into 3 subgroups, described below. Risk factors for the prevalence of underlying malignancy include, but are not limited to, large tumor size, associated mass, mural nodules, or thickened septal wall, eggshell calcification, and age [4].

MCNs usually lack the prominent extra cystic inflammatory component so characteristic of pancreatic pseudocysts.

Management

As with all forms of PCNs, surgical resection is indicated in cysts with positive cytology, associated complications, features concerning for malignancy, and cysts with significant malignant potential, including but not limited to MCNs. The choice of surgical technique depends largely on the size and location of the cyst, with lesions at the head of the pancreas requiring pancreaticoduodenectomy and lesions in the tail necessitating a distal pancreatectomy. A middle pancreatectomy can be considered for MCNs in the body of the pancreas.

In patients with an acceptable surgical risk, MCNs necessitate resection given their significant malignant potential. The majority of MCNs are found in the body and tail, therefore standard curative resection involves a distal pancreatectomy. Expert consensus suggests parenchymal-sparing resections and splenic preservation when possible, either via open or laparoscopic techniques. Lymphadenectomy is neither indicated nor beneficial. Intra-operatively, attention must be paid to remove the cyst intact so as to facilitate appropriate pathological examination and not rupture the cyst, spilling potentially malignant contents into the abdomen that could lead to tumor spread. Since spilling cyst contents could adversely affect the patient's outcome the surgeon should evaluate whether a laparoscopic or open operation would be safest.

Typical Findings of Mucinous Cystic Neoplasms [20]	
Age at presentation	Variable, usually 5th to 7th decade
Gender distribution	Almost exclusively female
Clinical presentation	Incidentally discovered, abdominal pain, or malignancy related
Imaging characteristics	Unilocular or septated cyst +/- wall calcifications; solid component, if present, may suggest malignancy
Aspirate characteristics	Viscous
Cytology findings	Columnar cells with variable atypia; stains positive for mucin; yield <50% but high yield from solid component for malignancy
CEA level	>200 ng/mL in approximately 75% of lesions
DNA analysis	K-ras mutation specific (>90%), not sensitive (<50%); high DNA amount or high-amplitude allelic loss seen in malignancy
Relative malignant potential	Moderate
Treatment	Resection

Mayo Clinic Histopathological Classification [7]		
Mucinous Cystadenomas	Contain uniform single layer of benign columnar mucinous cells	~65% of MCNs
Non-invasive, proliferative MCNs	Varying degree of atypia, dysplasia, Endothelial infolding and, carcinoma in situ in epithelial lining but *without* tissue invasion	~$30% of MCNs
Mucinous Cystadenocarcinomas	Overt stromal invasion beyond the epithelium	~5-10% of MCNs

Surgical resection is almost always curative for noninvasive MCNs. If successfully removed prior to transmural invasion, operative intervention portends a favorable prognosis with almost 100% survival [17]. Indeed in these patients detailed follow-up may be unnecessary given their "curative" resection [7]. For those with an associated invasive carcinoma, prognosis depends on the extent of invasion, stage, and resectability. The 2-year survival rate and 5-year survival rate of patients with resected MCN with an associated invasive carcinoma are about 67% and 50%, respectively [19]. If tissue invasion is present, adjuvant therapy should be considered even in cases of complete resection with no nodal metastasis.

In the case of lesions where diagnosis remains unclear despite a complete work-up, management depends on factors that increase the risk of malignancy. Resection is indicated in the case of positive cytology, a mucinous cyst ≥3 cm associated with main duct dilation and/or a definitive mural nodule, or KRAS and/or GNAS mutations with TP53 and PIK3CA or PTEN mutations by molecular testing [10]. For patients not meeting the above criteria, routine surveillance with MRI/MRCP is recommended at the one-year mark and then every 2 years for patients who remain surgical candidates. Any concerning changes in cyst characteristics or the development of symptoms attributable to the cyst should prompt repeat EUS-FNA.

For patients who are not surgical candidates or those who refuse an operation, it is reasonable to consider EUS-guided cyst ablation therapies.

References

[1] Sharma A. Tumors of the Pancreas. In: NJ Greenberger RB, R Burakoff, editor. Current Diagnosis & Treatment: *Gastroenterology, Hepatology, & Endoscopy*. McGraw-Hill, New York 2009. p. 318.

[2] Crippa S, Salvia R, Warshaw AL, Dominguez I, Bassi C, Falconi M, et al. Mucinous cystic neoplasm of the pancreas is not an aggressive entity: lessons from 163 resected patients. *Annals of surgery*. 2008;247(4):571-9. Epub 2008/03/26.

[3] Valsangkar NP, Morales-Oyarvide V, Thayer SP, Ferrone CR, Wargo JA, Warshaw AL, et al. 851 resected cystic tumors of the pancreas: a 33-year experience at the Massachusetts General Hospital. *Surgery*. 2012;152(3 Suppl 1):S4-12. Epub 2012/07/10.

[4] Sakorafas GH, Smyrniotis V, Reid-Lombardo KM, Sarr MG. Primary pancreatic cystic neoplasms revisited. Part III. Intraductal papillary mucinous neoplasms. *Surgical oncology*. 2011;20(2):e109-18. Epub 2011/03/15.

[5] Fernandez-del Castillo C, Targarona J, Thayer SP, Rattner DW, Brugge WR, Warshaw AL. Incidental pancreatic cysts: clinicopathologic characteristics and comparison with symptomatic patients. *Arch Surg*. 2003;138(4):427-3; discussion 33-4. Epub 2003/04/11.

[6] Gress F, Gottlieb K, Cummings O, Sherman S, Lehman G. Endoscopic ultrasound characteristics of mucinous cystic neoplasms of the pancreas. *The American journal of gastroenterology*. 2000;95(4):961-5. Epub 2000/04/14.

[7] Sarr MG, Carpenter HA, Prabhakar LP, Orchard TF, Hughes S, van Heerden JA, et al. Clinical and pathologic correlation of 84 mucinous cystic neoplasms of the pancreas: can one reliably differentiate benign from malignant (or premalignant) neoplasms? *Annals of surgery*. 2000;231(2):205-12. Epub 2000/02/16.

[8] Zamboni G, Scarpa A, Bogina G, Iacono C, Bassi C, Talamini G, et al. Mucinous cystic tumors of the pancreas: clinicopathological features, prognosis, and relationship to other mucinous cystic tumors. *The American journal of surgical pathology*. 1999;23(4):410-22. Epub 1999/04/13.

[9] Wilentz RE, Albores-Saavedra J, Zahurak M, Talamini MA, Yeo CJ, Cameron JL, et al. Pathologic examination accurately predicts prognosis in mucinous cystic neoplasms of the pancreas. *The American journal of surgical pathology*. 1999;23(11):1320-7. Epub 1999/11/11.

[10] Vege SS, Ziring B, Jain R, Moayyedi P. American gastroenterological association institute guideline on the diagnosis and management of asymptomatic neoplastic pancreatic cysts. *Gastroenterology*. 2015;148(4):819-22; quize12-3. Epub 2015/03/26.

[11] Brugge WR, Lewandrowski K, Lee-Lewandrowski E, Centeno BA, Szydlo T, Regan S, et al. Diagnosis of pancreatic cystic neoplasms: a

report of the cooperative pancreatic cyst study. *Gastroenterology*. 2004;126(5):1330-6. Epub 2004/05/08.

[12] Hutchins GF, Draganov PV. Cystic neoplasms of the pancreas: a diagnostic challenge. *World journal of gastroenterology*. 2009;15(1):48-54. Epub 2008/12/31.

[13] Khalid A, Zahid M, Finkelstein SD, LeBlanc JK, Kaushik N, Ahmad N, et al. Pancreatic cyst fluid DNA analysis in evaluating pancreatic cysts: a report of the PANDA study. *Gastrointestinal endoscopy*. 2009;69(6):1095-102. Epub 2009/01/21.

[14] Organization WH. Classification of Tumours. Pathology and Genetics of Tumours of the Digestive System. In: L.A. Aaltonen SRH, editor. Lyon, France *IARC Press*; 2000.

[15] Brugge WR, Lauwers GY, Sahani D, Fernandez-del Castillo C, Warshaw AL. Cystic neoplasms of the pancreas. *The New England journal of medicine*. 2004;351(12):1218-26. Epub 2004/09/17.

[16] Al-Haddad M, Gill KR, Raimondo M, Woodward TA, Krishna M, Crook JE, et al. Safety and efficacy of cytology brushings versus standard fine-needle aspiration in evaluating cystic pancreatic lesions: a controlled study. *Endoscopy*. 2010;42(2):127-32. Epub 2009/12/10.

[17] Sarr MG, Murr M, Smyrk TC, Yeo CJ, Fernandez-del-Castillo C, Hawes RH, et al. Primary cystic neoplasms of the pancreas. Neoplastic disorders of emerging importance-current state-of-the-art and unanswered questions. *Journal of gastrointestinal surgery : official journal of the Society for Surgery of the Alimentary Tract*. 2003;7(3):417-28. Epub 2003/03/26.

[18] Reddy RP, Smyrk TC, Zapiach M, Levy MJ, Pearson RK, Clain JE, et al. Pancreatic mucinous cystic neoplasm defined by ovarian stroma: demographics, clinical features, and prevalence of cancer. *Clinical gastroenterology and hepatology : the official clinical practice journal of the American Gastroenterological Association*. 2004;2(11):1026-31. Epub 2004/11/20.

[19] Yoon WJ, Brugge WR. Pancreatic cystic neoplasms: diagnosis and management. *Gastroenterology clinics of North America.* 2012;41(1):103-18. Epub 2012/02/22.

[20] Khalid A, Brugge W. ACG practice guidelines for the diagnosis and management of neoplastic pancreatic cysts. *The American journal of gastroenterology*. 2007;102(10):2339-49. Epub 2007/09/04.

In: Cystic Tumors of the Pancreas
Editor: Robert Grützmann

ISBN: 978-1-53612-523-8

Chapter 11

Rare Cystic Tumors of the Pancreas

Ulrich Friedrich Wellner, MD, PhD and Tobias Keck, MD, PhD, MBA, FACS
Clinic of Surgery, UKSH Campus Lübeck, Lübeck, Germany

Abstract

Besides intraductal papillary mucinous neoplasm, serous cystic adenoma and mucinous cystic neoplasm, there are several rare neoplasms that also can appear as a cystic tumor of the pancreas. Although these entities are very rare, physicians practicing in centers for pancreatology and pancreatic surgery are likely to encounter patients with these diseases in practice. There are several specific features characterizing most of these rare tumors, which can be helpful in diagnosis and planning of treatment. Improved imaging as well as case series and reviews thereof contributed significantly to provide more and clinically relevant data on these tumors over the past decade.

Keywords: cystic neoplasm of the pancreas, cystic tumor of the pancreas, solid pseudopapillary neoplasm, pancreatic surgery

SPN Solid Pseudopapillary Neoplasm

Solid-pseudopapillary neoplasm (SPN) is a rare tumor of the pancreas, which due to its frequently cystic appearance, is often mentioned among the cystic neoplasms of the pancreas (CNP). However, SPN can also have mixed solid and cystic as well as totally solid appearance in preoperative imaging (Figure 1) [1]. A peculiar histopathologic feature of SPN is its nuclear expression of E-Cadherin. The first description of an SPN is credited to AO Whipple's collegue Frantz [2], and some authors refer to it by the name Frantz tumor. Other inconsistent nomenclature was applied, until the WHO classification officially adopted the name SPN [3].

The most specific clinical feature of SPN is probably its typical occurrence in young women: a current review of all published cases since the 1950s shows that 88% of patients with SPN were female, with a mean age at diagnosis of 29 years. Unlike mucinous cystic neoplasm of the pancreas (MCN), which also has a predominance in women, SPN arise throughout the whole pancreas. Detection of SPN seems to have increased during the last decade, which is probably the result of increased use of modern cross-sectional imaging, resulting in >90% of all SPN reported since the 1950s being reported in the past 15 years. The most common presentation is with unspecific abdominal complaints, while only about 10% of patients present with jaundice, pancreatitis or weight loss and 10% are incidental findings. Observational data suggests that computed tomography and magnetic resonance imaging are the best means to diagnose SPN, while endoscopic ultrasound and fine-needle aspiration yield relatively low diagnostic accuracy.

The standard of care is surgical resection. SPN can be considered a semi-malignant neoplasm with invasive local growth but rare metastasis. In the absence of clear signs of lymphatic spread, resection can be performed by parenchyma-preserving resections, as the incidence of lymph node metastasis is only 2%. Data on adjuvant treatment is scarce, because there is usually no indication. The rate of recurrence or distant metastasis is in the range of 5%. However, recurrence typically occurs with considerable delay (mean over 4 years), warranting long-term postoperative surveillance [1].

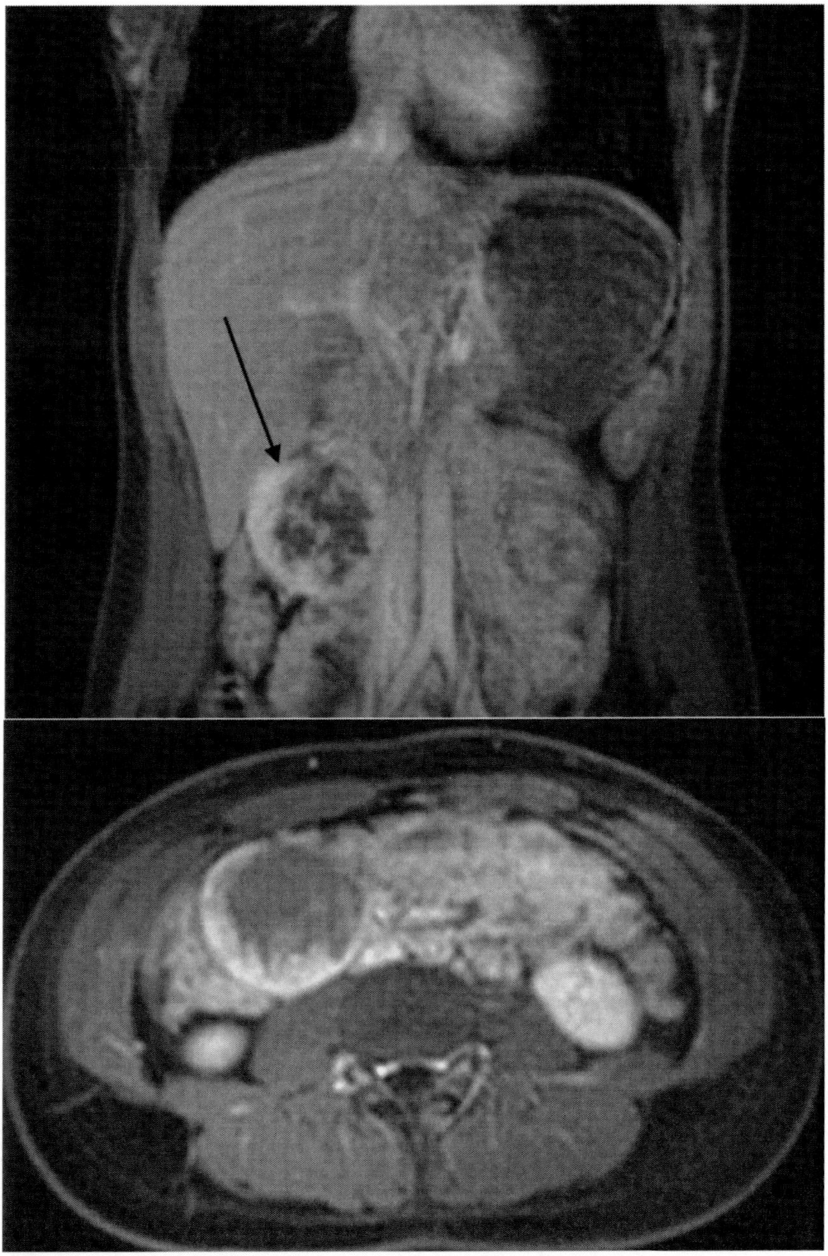

Figure 1. Magnetic resonance imaging demonstrating mixed solid and cystic appearance of a large asymptomatic solid pseudopapillary neoplasm in a 17-year old female. Pancreatoduodenectomy was curative.

Cystic Pancreatic Neuroendocrine Neoplasm (CPNEN)

CPNEN are a very rare form of cystic pancreatic neoplasm, with the first report credited to Thigpen in 1940 [4]. This entity has been reported to make up about 12% of all resected pancreatic neuroendocrine neoplasms (PNEN) [5]. While PNEN typically are solid, cystic growth seems to be an inherent feature of CPNEN, as the available evidence does not support a role of tumor necrosis or hemorrhage in the formation of the cystic component.

Preoperative diagnosis of CPNEN poses considerable challenges, and reported diagnostic accuracy is only about 50-60%. EUS-guided fine-needle aspiration and cytology might be the most reliable diagnostic means, but remain operator-dependent. Paralleling the hyperdense appearance of PNEN in contrast-enhanced computed tomography, CPNEN may be distinguished by a rim enhancement derived from hyper-vascularization. When compared to their solid counterparts, CPNEN seem to have a slightly less aggressive biology. Despite a larger size on average, CPNEN display a lower rate of lymph node metastasis, vascular invasion, mitotic count or Ki67 proliferation index. Likewise, several comparative studies reported increased disease-free and overall survival in patients with CPNEN compared to PNEN [5].

Lack of data on observation versus resection as well as reliable diagnostic tools preclude specific recommendations on therapy of CPNEN. Therefore, in case of preoperative diagnosis of a CPNEN, the guidelines for treatment of PNEN might be followed [6].

Intraductal Tubular Neoplasm

Intraductal tubular neoplasm (ITN) is characterized by intraductal growth of neoplastic epithelium with variable degree of dysplasia [7]. Clinically and morphologically, it shows many parallels to intraductal papillary mucinous neoplasm (IPMN), but the distinguishing feature is tubular growth of the neoplastic epithelium with pyloric gland differentiation and occasional goblet cells. The typical immunohistochemical profile is positive for CK7, CK19, MUC5A and MUC6, and negative for CK20, CDX2, MUC1 and MUC2. As carcinoma in situ (intraductal tubular carcinoma) and invasive growth are present in a considerable (30-60%) proportion of resected cases, resection remains the treatment of choice.

CYSTIC ACINAR NEOPLASMS

Neoplasia with pancreatic acinar differentiation is very rare, and can display cystic growth. These lesions can have benign (acinar cystadenoma, ACA) or malignant (acinar cystadenocarcinoma ACAC) nature [7]. Histologically, the cysts are lined with single or multiple layers of epithelium with acinar differentiation, displaying PAS-positive granules and immunohistochemical staining for pancreatic enzymes (Lipase, Trypsin, Chymotrypsin). Interestingly, the neoplastic cells also stain positive for Cytokeratin 7, which is considered a marker of pancreatic ductal epithelium. In ACAC, there are signs of epithelial dysplasia and occasionally prominent intraductal growth, as well as invasion and metastasis.

Due to the limited number of reported cases, no recommendations on preoperative diagnostic features can be given. The treatment of choice seems to be radical resection. Prognosis after resection of ACAC has been reported to be slightly better than in non-cystic pancreatic acinar adenocarcinoma as well as pancreatic ductal adenocarcinoma.

CYSTIC PANCREATOBLASTOMA

Pancreatoblastoma is the most frequent pancreatic neoplasm in children in the first decade of life, but nevertheless is very rare, with less than 100 cases reported in the literature [7]. While the solid subtype is more common, the cystic pancreatoblastoma is usually associated with Beckwidth-Wiedemann Syndrome. The latter is characterized by macrosomia, visceromegalia, omphalocele, macroglossia and an elevated risk (4%) to develop embryonal tumors. Most patients are asymptomatic. On imaging, the tumor usually appears as a large solid lesion compressing rather than invading adjacent organs. Local or distant metastasis is observed in about one third of patients at diagnosis. Radical resection is the treatment of choice, and in the absence of metastasis, prognosis seems to be good. Adjuvant therapy has been used empirically but its role remains undefined.

Cystic Degeneration of Solid Pancreatic Malignancy

Several solid pancreatic malignancies have been reported to have cystic components in rare cases. The mechanisms responsible for cystic degeneration usually result in a mixed solid and cystic morphology. Pancreatic ductal adenocarcinoma (PDAC) typically causes stenosis with increased intraductal pressure and proximal dilatation of the pancreatic duct. This can result in the formation of so-called retention cysts in the associated non-neoplastic parts of the pancreas. Furthermore, PDAC can cause acute pancreatitis with pancreatic tissue necrosis and subsequent cyst formation. Another mechanism of cyst formation is tumor necrosis resulting from disturbed nutrition and oxygen supply, as typically observed in large, fast-growing poorly differentiated PDAC. Cystic degeneration has also been reported in the large-duct, adenosquamous and undifferentiated carcinoma with osteoclast-like giant cells subtypes of pancreatic cancer. Furthermore, mucinous cystic adenocarcinoma may result from malignant degeneration of mucinous cystic neoplasm (MCN) (Figure 2, see Chapter on MCN). Definite preoperative diagnosis is seldom achieved and only possible by biopsy. Radical resection is the treatment of choice, but prognosis remains poor.

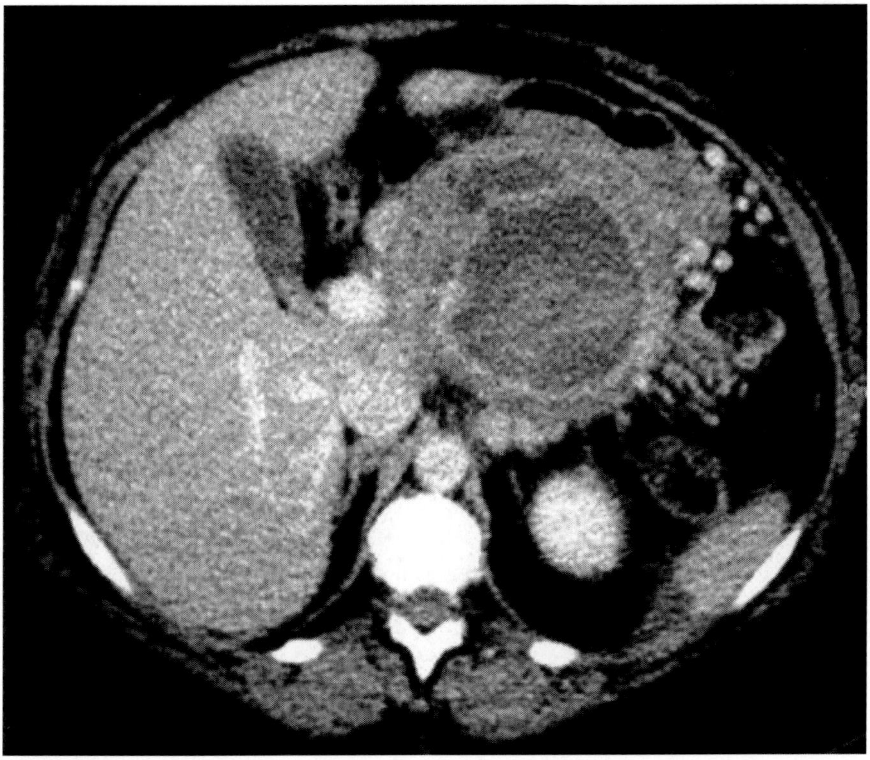

Figure 2. Large mucinous cystadenocarcinoma of the pancreas in a 42-year old female in contrast-enhanced computed tomography. The tumor had been mistaken as a pancreatic pseudocyst for about 15 years and became symptomatic by arrosion into the large bowel and bleeding. Curative resection was not feasible at the time of diagnosis.

Cystic Degeneration of Metastasis to the Pancreas

As with primary pancreatic malignancy, metastases to the pancreas have been observed to display mixed solid and cystic appearance. Renal cell carcinoma is the most frequently reported primary tumor in these cases. Of note, preoperative diagnosis of pancreatic metastasis is usually possible on the basis of history, imaging and FNA, and prognosis after resection of renal cell carcinoma metastases is much better than for primary pancreatic malignancy [8].

Cystic Germ Cell Tumors

Extragonadal pancreatic germ cell tumors are extraordinarily rare. Few cases of choriocarcinoma and mature cystic teratoma have been described [7]. The latter is most frequently observed in young adults and often grows to considerable size before diagnosis. Preoperative diagnosis is usually not possible and resection is the treatment of choice.

Cystic Mesenchymal Tumors

Tumors arising from mesenchymal tissue can occur anywhere in the body. Some have been reported to form cystic tumors in the pancreas, but are exceedingly rare [7]. Among these are inflammatory myofibroblastic neoplasm, extragastrointestinal stromal neoplasm, solitary fibrous neoplasm, and Schwannoma. The latter are associated with von Recklinghausen disease (Neurofibromatosis), where malignant transformation can occur in about 10%. Resection in the absence of malignancy is curative and can be achieved by enucleation.

Pancreatic Cystic Hamartoma

Pancreatic hamartomas are very rare non-neoplastic lesions that may appear cystic on imaging [7]. Diagnosis is usually made only after resection.

Pancreatic Lymphoepithelial Cyst

Lymphoepithelial cyst of the pancreas (PLEC) is a very rare condition, of which only roughly over 100 cases have been published since the 1980s [9]. Histologically, PLEC is characterized by a mature squamous epithelial lining, surrounded by lymphatic tissue with follicles, and filled with keratinous debris. Three hypotheses of the pathogenesis have been suggested: ectopic branchial cleft from embyogenesis, inclusion of benign epithelium in a pancreatic lymph node and squamous metaplasia of obstructed pancreatic ducts.

A current review of the literature demonstrates that about 40% of patients report abdominal pain, while another roughly 40% of PLEC are incidental findings. Median patient age is 55 years and there is a male predominance (about 80%). The distribution over the pancreas seems homogenous.

As not a single case of metastasis or recurrence has been reported, so theoretically the disease could be managed conservatively in the absence of symptoms. However, diagnostic accuracy is much too low to allow for this approach: Imaging suggests PLEC in only 20%, and even FNA is diagnostic in only 40%. In addition, over 50% of patients have elevations in serum CA19.9 (median ca. 130 U/ml), and also CA19.9 and CEA levels in cystic fluid are typically elevated, with occasional extreme levels, leading to resection for suspected malignancy. With regard to the reported cases, conservative management was pursued in about 10%, while 40% were radically resected and 40% revecived limited resections.

CYSTIC LYMPHANGIOMA

Cystic lymphangioma is considered a non-neoplastic lesion arising by obstructed lymphatic flow due to congenital anomalies of the local lymphatic system [7]. Histologically, the cystic space is lines by lymphatic endothelium negative for Cytokeratin. The lesions are most often located in the pancreatic tail region. They may not directly involve the pancreatic parenchyma as they arise from retroperitoneal lymphatics. Most patients are asymptomatic and imaging shows a multiloculated water-isodense cystic mass in the retroperitoneum. Resection is usually required to establish the diagnosis (Figure 3). Complete resection is curative, but recurrence can occur after incomplete resection.

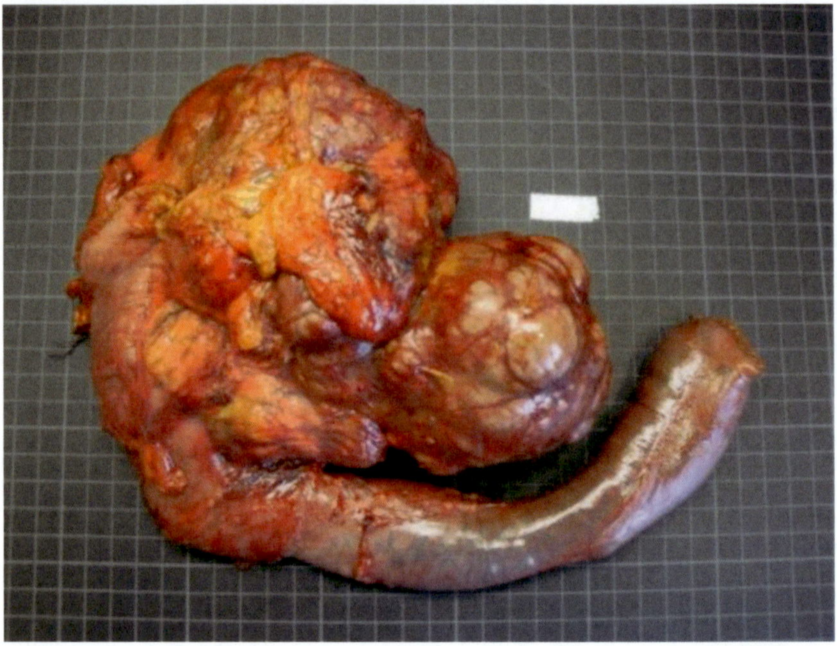

Figure 3. Pancreatoduodenectomy resection specimen of a large lymphangioma in the pancreatic head. Diagnosis was established only after histopathological workup.

Cavernous Hemangioma

These benign tumors consist of dilated vascular channels and therefore also appear cystic [7]. Women are more frequently affected and there is an association with von Hippel Lindau syndrome. Imaging with intravenous contrast can reveal the diagnosis. Resection is only necessary for symptomatic or rapidly enlarging lesions.

Pancreatic Tuberculosis

Pancreatic tuberculosis may present as solid or cystic mass with associated lymphadenopathy, mimicking pancreatic cancer or cystic neoplasms (Figure 4) [10]. Pancreatic tuberculosis is rare even in patients with tuberculosis, where it is reported in only 2-5% of cases in autopsy series. Antimycobacterial effects of pancreatic extracts as well as enzymes have been observed and offered as an explanation. Three types of pancreatic tuberculosis are recognized: diffuse involvement in the form of military tuberculosis, affection from peripancreatic lymph nodes, and localized pancreatic tuberculosis.

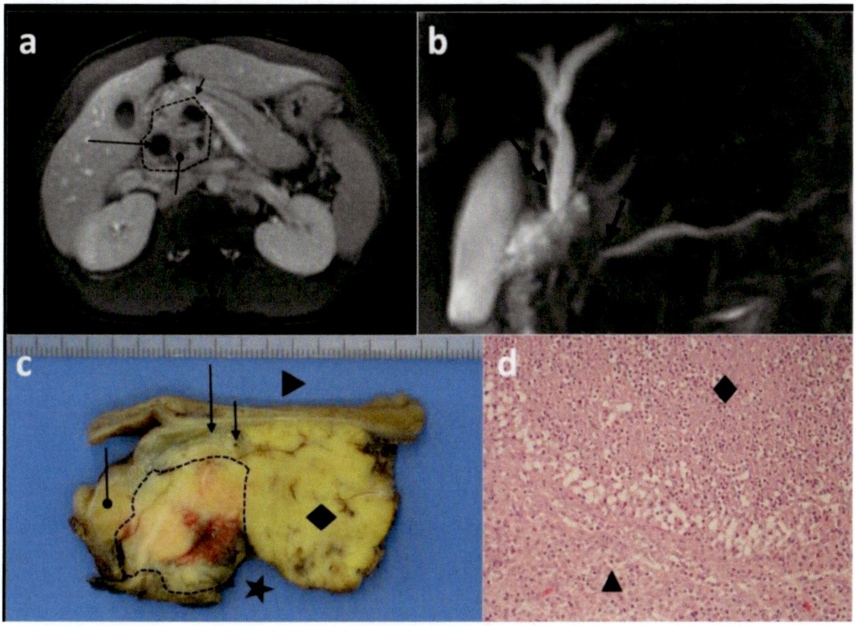

Figure 4. Pancreatic tuberculosis mimicking a cystic pancreatic head tumor. a) Contrast-enhanced MRI shows a mass of the pancreatic head (encircled) with solid (blunt arrow) and cystic (arrow) areas, irregular enhancement in the solid portion and the cystic wall, heterogeneous signal intensity as well as areas of high intensity corresponding to hemorrhage and a severely compressed and possibly infiltrated portal vein. b) MRCP discloses a slight compression and dilatation (long arrow) of the distal bile duct. Of note, the pancreatic duct does not show signs of obstruction (short arrow). Pancreatoduodenectomy with en-bloc portal venous resection was performed for suspected malignancy. c) macroscopic section through the formalin-fixed pancreatoduodenectomy specimen, square: pancreatic head, triangle: duodenum, encircled: area of massive caseating granulomatous inflammation, asterisk: portal venous resection margin, long arrow: compressed bile duct, short arrow: pancreatic duct, blunt arrow: enlarged peripancreatic lymph node. d) histopathological workup demonstrates massive granulomatous inflammation (triangle mark) and caseating necrosis (square mark).

Most cases are reported in patients from the Indian subcontinent and Southeast Asia, where tuberculosis continues to be a major public health problem. Presentation is usually with unspecific abdominal complaints, often associated with other symptoms of tuberculosis like fever, night sweat and weight loss, while obstructive jaundice is very seldom. Cross-sectional imaging can reveal solid, cystic or mixed masses and abscess, as well as lymphadenopathy or even vascular involvement. Therefore, differentiation from pancreatic cancer or cystic neoplasms by imaging alone is often not possible. A distinctive feature might be that the pancreatic and the bile duct are rarely obstructed and dilated, even with large mass forming lesions in the pancreatic head.

Key to preoperative diagnosis is usually a history of tuberculosis or typical symptoms thereof. EUS-guided FNA can help establish the diagnosis by demonstration of granulomatous inflammation, acid-fast rods, and identification of Mycobacterium tuberculosis by culture or polymerase chain reaction (PCR). In the absence of these diagnostic clues, surgical tissue biopsy is needed.

Due to the diagnostic difficulties, some case series and reviews report radical pancreatic resections performed for pancreatic tuberculosis. Surgical treatment is however not considered necessary, as pancreatic tuberculosis can usually be healed with standard tuberculostatic medication.

References

[1] Law JK, Ahmed A, Singh VK, Akshintala VS, Olson MT, Raman SP, et al. A Systematic Review of Solid-Pseudopapillary Neoplasms: Are these rare lesions? *Pancreas.* 2014 Apr;43(3):331–7.

[2] Frantz V. Tumors of the pancreas. In: *Atlas of Tumor Pathology*. Washington DC, USA: US Armed Forces Institute of Pathology; 1959. p. 32–3. (1st series).

[3] Bosman FT, Carneiro F, Hruban RH, Theise ND. WHO classification of tumors of the digestive system. 4th edition. Lyon, France: *International Agency for Research in Cancer;* 2010. (WHO classification of tumors).

[4] Singhi AD, Chu LC, Tatsas AD, Shi C, Ellison TA, Fishman EK, et al. Cystic pancreatic neuroendocrine tumors: a clinicopathologic study. *Am J Surg Pathol.* 2012 Nov;36(11):1666–73.

[5] Koh Y-X, Chok A-Y, Zheng H-L, Tan C-S, Goh BKP. A systematic review and meta-analysis of the clinicopathologic characteristics of cystic versus solid pancreatic neuroendocrine neoplasms. *Surgery.* 2014 Mar 18.

[6] Salazar R, Wiedenmann B, Rindi G, Ruszniewski P. ENETS 2011 Consensus Guidelines for the Management of Patients with Digestive Neuroendocrine Tumors: an update. *Neuroendocrinology.* 2012;95(2):71–3.

[7] Sakorafas GH, Smyrniotis V, Reid-Lombardo KM, Sarr MG. Primary pancreatic cystic neoplasms of the pancreas revisited. Part IV: rare cystic neoplasms. *Surg Oncol.* 2012 Sep;21(3):153–63.

[8] Chang Y-H, Liaw C-C, Chuang C-K. The role of surgery in renal cell carcinoma with pancreatic metastasis. *Biomed J.* 2015 Apr;38(2):173–6.

[9] Mege D, Grégoire E, Barbier L, Del Grande J, Le Treut YP. Lymphoepithelial cyst of the pancreas: an analysis of 117 patients. *Pancreas*. 2014 Oct;43(7):987–95.

[10] Chaudhary P, Bhadana U, Arora MP. Pancreatic Tuberculosis. *Indian J Surg.* 2015 Dec;77(6):517–24.

SECTION VII. FOLLOW-UP

In: Cystic Tumors of the Pancreas
Editor: Robert Grützmann
ISBN: 978-1-53612-523-8

Chapter 12

SURVEILLANCE AND FOLLOW-UP OF CYSTIC TUMORS

Takayuki Anazawa, MD, PhD, Kyoichi Takaori*, MD, PhD, Toshihiko Masui, MD, PhD and Shinji Uemoto, MD, PhD

Division of Hepato-Biliary-Pancreatic Surgery and Transplantation, Department of Surgery, Graduate School of Medicine, Kyoto University, Kyoto, Japan

ABSTRACT

With the increased use of diagnostic imaging, the opportunities for the detection of pancreatic cystic tumors are increasing. Several guidelines were proposed for the management of these cysts. However, recommendations on surveillance and surgical resection were based on low-quality evidence. We reviewed the current surveillance methods for pancreatic cystic tumors including IPMN, MCN, and others based on the existing guidelines.

Keywords: IPMN, MCN, surveillance, EUS

* Corresponding Author Email: takaori@kuhp.kyoto-u.ac.jp.

INTRODUCTION

With the increased use of diagnostic imaging, the opportunities for the detection of pancreatic cystic tumors are increasing. Computed tomography (CT) and magnetic resonance imaging (MRI) studies have indicated that the prevalence of pancreatic cysts is approximately 2.5% in the general population [1, 2] and increases with age. Many cysts are consistent with small, branch-duct (BD) intraductal papillary mucinous neoplasms (IPMNs). Most of these are benign, but some cases of BD-IPMN, main-duct IPMN, mucinous cystic neoplasm (MCN), and solid pseudopapillary tumor (SPT) have malignant potential. The natural history and predictive factors of malignant alterations in these tumors have not yet been elucidated, and optimal surveillance or follow-up procedures have not been established. Several guidelines were proposed by medical societies and experts for the management of these cysts [3-5]. However, recommendations on surveillance and surgical resection were based on low-quality evidence. In this chapter, we review the surveillance methods of pancreatic cystic tumors including IPMN, MCN, and others based on the existing guidelines and attempt to address issues for future discussion.

SURVEILLANCE OF NON-RESECTED IPMN

The American Gastroenterological Association (AGA) Guidelines recommend surveillance of cystic tumors using MRI [6]. An MRI is recommended in the beginning, at 1 year, and every 2 years thereafter, regardless of the size of the tumor. In a consensus statement by European experts, follow-up with either EUS or MRI is recommended, and the initial follow-up is done every 6 months, after 1 year, and every year thereafter, regardless of the size of the tumor [7]. However, the International Association of Pancreatology (IAP) consensus guidelines, also called the Fukuoka Guidelines, recommend surveillance methods based on the cyst diameter [4]. Figure 1 shows the outline.

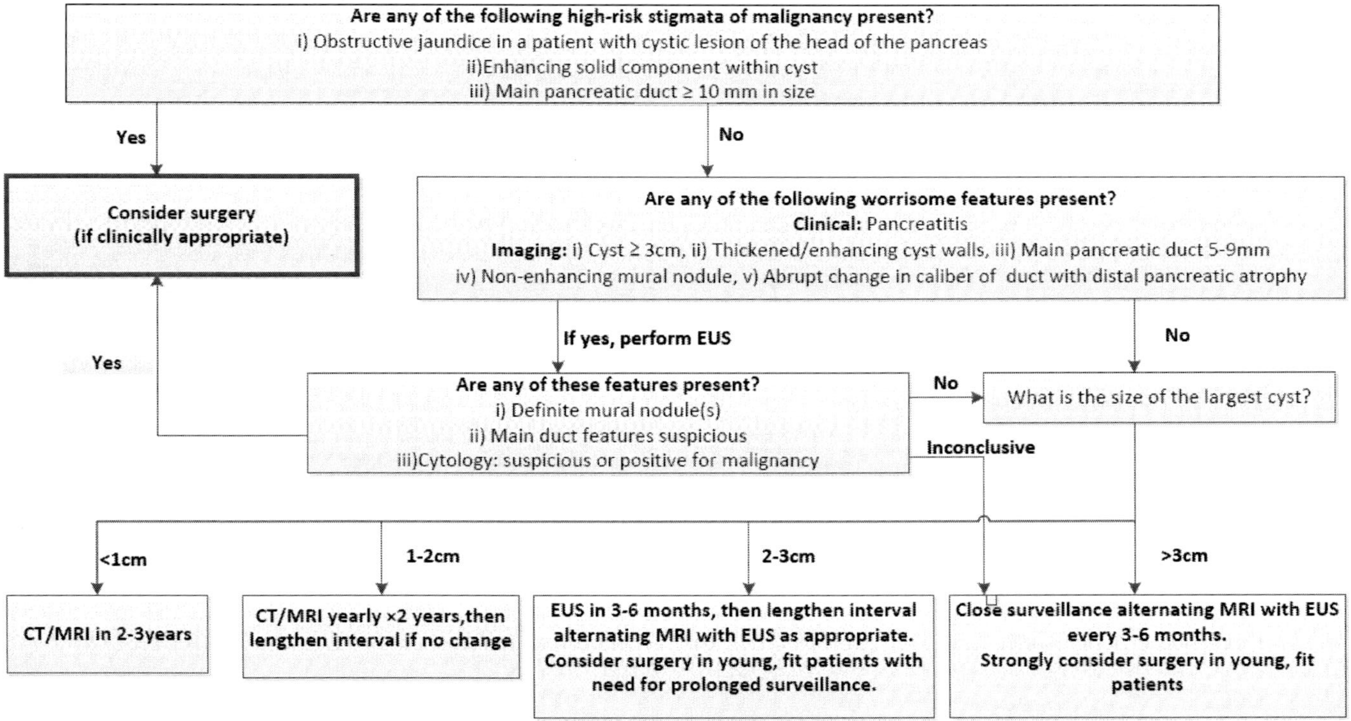

Figure 1. The Fukuoka guidelines for managing patients presumed to have BD-IPMN.

For tumors with a cyst diameter of 3 cm or more, or those with worrisome features but no evidence of malignancy, close surveillance alternating MRI with EUS every 3–6 months are recommended. If the cyst diameter is 2–3 cm, EUS or MRI is performed every 3–6 months, and if the cyst diameter is less than 2 cm, it is recommended to perform CT or MRI once a year. If the cyst diameter is less than 3 cm and if there is no change in the medical condition, an extension of the examination interval may be considered. If the expertise is available, EUS with cytopathology [8], CEA [9], and molecular analyses [10] may be considered. Mukewar et al., validated the risk stratification proposed in the Fukuoka guidelines [11]. They estimated the 5-year risk of pancreatic cancer in Fukuoka-positive (high-risk or worrisome features) and Fukuoka-negative (no high-risk or worrisome features) cysts and concluded that the Fukuoka Guidelines allow risk stratification of cysts for pancreatic cancer. Nevertheless, the overall risk of pancreatic cancer is low in Fukuoka-negative and Fukuoka-positive cysts with worrisome features beyond the 6-month follow-up period. It remains difficult to determine the appropriate surveillance strategies based on morphological criteria. It is expected that future studies on molecular markers of malignant IPMNs will provide us with a more accurate diagnosis and better surveillance strategies.

Follow-Up of Surgically Resected IPMN and MCN

IPMN requires long-term follow-up as there is a risk of IPMN recurrence and subsequent pancreatic cancer development due to residual tumor tissue, even after resection. Recurrence has been reported in 5%–10% of resected non-invasive IPMNs [7]. Based on the Fukuoka Guidelines, surveillance recommendations have been stated for three cases: i) a known BD-IPMN left unresected, ii) development of new lesions in the remnant pancreas, and/or iii) residual IPMN detected in the surgical margins [4]. In cases of known IPMN in the remnant pancreas, patients should be followed as non-resected IPMNs. In case i), patients should be followed as non-resected IPMNs. In case ii), if no residual lesions are observed and the margins are negative, repeat examinations at 2 and 5 years may be reasonable. Case iii) is more complex. The resection margin may show normal pancreatic tissue, non-dysplastic changes, low-grade dysplasia, moderate-grade dysplasia, high-grade dysplasia, or invasive carcinoma [12]. If the margin shows normal pancreatic tissue or non-dysplastic changes, patients should be followed as non-resected cases. If the margin shows low-grade or moderate-grade dysplasia, Fukuoka Guidelines suggest that patient history/physical examination and MRCP be performed twice a year. However, the AGA Guidelines suggest against routine surveillance of pancreatic cysts without high-grade dysplasia or invasive carcinoma after surgical resection [6], except in mixed-duct IPMN and if there is a strong family history of pancreatic cancer, because there are some concerns regarding possible development of invasive cancer in the remnant pancreas. The AGA suggests that even the patient with resected invasive carcinoma in a cystic lesion should undergo MRI surveillance every 2 years. The consensus statement of the European experts suggests a yearly follow-up using non-radiating (MRI or EUS) imaging. Neither of these recommendations are based on high-quality evidence.

MCNs are usually solitary and potentially malignant, but complete resection of a non-invasive MCN is curative. In such cases, no routine surveillance is needed after resection [4, 7]. The rate of development of invasive carcinoma from MCNs has been reported to be 12%–20% [13, 14], and the invasive MCNs show a similar pathological phenotype as invasive ductal adenocarcinoma. Accordingly, patients who have undergone resection for invasive MCNs should receive follow-up surveillance in the same manner as a pancreatic cancer patient.

Surveillance of Other Pancreatic Cysts

The majority of serous cyst neoplasms (SCNs) are benign. Clinically significant symptoms are rare; tumor growth rate is slow, and the influence on the patient's lifespan is very small. Therefore, if a patient is diagnosed with SCN, there is no indication for surgery, except in symptomatic or malignant SCNs, which are extremely rare [15]. When SCN is suspected, careful evaluation using CT, MRI, and EUS is necessary. Non-resected patients may enter a follow-up program, initially repeated after 3–6 months and then with further intervals depending on tumor growth rate [7], especially when other potentially malignant neoplasms are also suspected.

Solid pseudopapillary neoplasms (SPNs) have malignant potential, and accordingly, surgical resection is the treatment of choice for SPNs. In order to prevent local recurrence, dissemination, and recurrence in lymph nodes, extensive resection with negative surgical margins is necessary for the treatment of SPN [16]. The prognosis after resection is good, and it has been reported that the 5-year survival rate after resection is 95% or more [17, 18]. Relapse after resection has been reported in approximately 4% of cases [19]. On average, the time to recurrence is 4 years or more, and a follow-up of at least 5 years after resection is recommended.

References

[1] Laffan, T. A., Horton, K. M., Klein, A. P., Berlanstein, B., Siegelman, S. S., Kawamoto, S., Johnson, P. T., Fishman, E.K. and Hruban, R. H. (2008). Prevalence of unsuspected pancreatic cysts on MDCT. *AJR Am. J. Roentgenol.*, 191 (III): 802-807.

[2] de Jong, K., Nio, C. Y., Mearadji, B., Phoa, S. S., Engelbrecht, M. R., Dijkgraaf, M. G., Bruno, M. J. and Fockens, P. (2012). Disappointing interobserver agreement among radiologists for a classifying diagnosis of pancreatic cysts using magnetic resonance imaging. *Pancreas*, 41 (II): 278-282.

[3] Tanaka, M., Chari, S., Adsay, V., Fernandez-del Castillo, C., Falconi, M., Shimizu, M., Yamaguchi, K., Yamao K., Matsuno, S. and International Association of Pancreatology (2006). International consensus guidelines for management of intraductal papillary

mucinous neoplasms and mucinous cystic neoplasms of the pancreas. *Pancreatology*, 6 (I-II): 17-32.

[4] Tanaka, M., Fernández-del Castillo, C., Adsay, V., Chari, S., Falconi, M., Jang, J. Y., Kimura, W., Levy, P., Pitman, M. B., Schmidt, C. M., Shimizu, M., Wolfgang, C. L., Yamaguchi, K., Yamao, K. and International Association of Pancreatology (2012). International consensus guidelines 2012 for the management of IPMN and MCN of the pancreas. *Pancreatology*, 12 (III): 183-197.

[5] Scheiman, J. M., Hwang, J. H. and Moayyedi, P. (2015). American gastroenterological association technical review on the diagnosis and management of asymptomatic neoplastic pancreatic cysts. *Gastroenterology*, 148 (IV): 824-848.e22.

[6] Vege, S. S., Ziring, B., Jain, R., Moayyedi, P., Committee C. G. and Association, A. G. (2015). American gastroenterological association institute guideline on the diagnosis and management of asymptomatic neoplastic pancreatic cysts. *Gastroenterology*, 148 (IV): 819-822; quize 12-13.

[7] Del Chiaro, M., Verbeke, C., Salvia, R., Klöppel, G., Werner, J., McKay, C., Friess, H., Manfredi, R., Van Cutsem, E., Löhr, M., Segersvärd, R. and European Study Group on Cystic Tumours of the Pancreaset (2013). European experts consensus statement on cystic tumors of the pancreas. *Dig. Liver Dis.*, 45 (IX): 703-711.

[8] Schmidt, C. M, White, P. B., Waters, J. A., Yiannoutsos, C. T., Cummings, O. W., Baker, M., Howard, T. J., Zyromski, N. J., Nakeeb, A., DeWitt J. M., Akisik, F. M., Sherman, S., Pitt, H.A. and Lillemoe, K. D. (2007). Intraductal papillary mucinous neoplasms: predictors of malignant and invasive pathology. *Ann. Surg.*, 246 (IV): 644-651; discussion 51-54.

[9] Cizginer, S., Turner, B. G., Turner, B., Bilge, A. R., Karaca, C., Pitman, M. B. and Brugge, W. R. (2011). Cyst fluid carcinoembryonic antigen is an accurate diagnostic marker of pancreatic mucinous cysts. *Pancreas*, 40 (VII): 1024-1028.

[10] Khalid, A., Zahid, M., Finkelstein, S. D., LeBlanc, J. K., Kaushik, N., Ahmad, N., Brugge, W. R., Edmundowicz, S. A., Hawes, R. H. and

McGrath, K. M. (2009). Pancreatic cyst fluid DNA analysis in evaluating pancreatic cysts: a report of the PANDA study. *Gastrointest. Endosc.,* 69 (VI): 1095-1102.

[11] Mukewar, S., de Pretis, N., Aryal-Khanal, A., Ahmed, N., Sah, R., Enders, F., Larson, J. J., Levy, M.J., Takahashi, N., Topazian, M. and Pearson, R. (2016) Fukuoka criteria accurately predict risk for adverse outcomes during follow-up of pancreatic cysts presumed to be intraductal papillary mucinous neoplasms. *Gut.*

[12] Couvelard, A., Sauvanet, A., Kianmanesh, R., Hammel, P., Colnot, N., Lévy, P., Ruszniewski, P., Bedossa, P. and Belghiti, J. (2005) Frozen sectioning of the pancreatic cut surface during resection of intraductal papillary mucinous neoplasms of the pancreas is useful and reliable: a prospective evaluation. *Ann. Surg*., 242 (VI): 774-778, discussion 8-80.

[13] Crippa, S., Salvia, R., Warshaw, A. L., Domínguez, I., Bassi, C., Falconi, M., Thayer, S. P., Zamboni, G., Lauwers, G. Y., Mino-Kenudson, M., Capelli, P., Pederzoli, P. and Castillo, C. F. (2008). Mucinous cystic neoplasm of the pancreas is not an aggressive entity: lessons from 163 resected patients. *Ann. Surg*., 247 (IV):571-579.

[14] Goh, B. K., Tan, Y. M., Chung, Y. F., Chow, P. K., Cheow, P. C., Wong, W. K. and Ooi, L. L. (2006) A review of mucinous cystic neoplasms of the pancreas defined by ovarian-type stroma: clinicopathological features of 344 patients. *World J. Surg*., 30 (XII): 2236-2245.

[15] Jais, B., Rebours, V., Malleo, G., Salvia, R., Fontana, M., Maggino, L., Bassi, C., Manfredi, R., Moran, R., Lennon, A. M. and Zaheer, A. (2016). Serous cystic neoplasm of the pancreas: a multinational study of 2622 patients under the auspices of the International Association of Pancreatology and European Pancreatic Club (European Study Group on Cystic Tumors of the Pancreas). *Gut*, 65 (II): 305-312.

[16] Vassos, N., Agaimy, A., Klein, P., Hohenberger, W. and Croner, R. S. (2013). Solid-pseudopapillary neoplasm (SPN) of the pancreas: case series and literature review on an enigmatic entity. *Int. J. Clin. Exp. Pathol.*, 6 (VI): 1051-1059.

[17] Tang, L. H., Aydin, H., Brennan, M. F. and Klimstra, D. S. (2005). Clinically aggressive solid pseudopapillary tumors of the pancreas: a report of two cases with components of undifferentiated carcinoma and a comparative clinicopathologic analysis of 34 conventional cases. *Am. J. Surg. Pathol.,* 29 (IV): 512-519.

[18] Martin, R. C., Klimstra, D. S., Brennan, M. F. and Conlon, K. C. (2002). Solid-pseudopapillary tumor of the pancreas: a surgical enigma? *Ann. Surg. Oncol.* 9 (I): 35-40.

[19] Law, J. K., Ahmed, A., Singh, V. K., Akshintala, V. S., Olson, M. T., Raman, S. P., Ali, S. Z., Fishman, E. K., Kamel, I., Canto, M.I. and Dal Molin, M. (2014). A systematic review of solid-pseudopapillary neoplasms: are these rare lesions? *Pancreas*, 43 (III): 331-337.

SECTION VIII. CLINICAL

In: Cystic Tumors of the Pancreas
Editor: Robert Grützmann
ISBN: 978-1-53612-523-8

Chapter 13

CLINICAL EXAMPLES

Stephan Kersting*[*], MD, PhD and Robert Grützmann, MD, PhD, MBA
Department of Surgery, University Hospital of Erlangen,
Friedrich-Alexander-University Erlangen-Nürnberg,
Erlangen, Germany

ABSTRACT

While cystic tumors of the pancreas can be difficult to distinguish in preoperative imaging, they still show certain characteristic features upon laparotomy or in the concluding stages of analyzing the surgical specimen. This chapter shows typical examples of the different cystic tumors in preoperative imaging, *in situ* and the final surgical specimen.

Keywords: pancreas, cystic tumors, clinical examples

[*] Corresponding Author: Email: stephan.kersting@uk-erlangen.de.

Introduction

Even for experienced clinicians, the differential diagnosis of cystic tumors of the pancreas is often difficult. However, the clinical distinction using information from CT- or MRI-scans, endosonography and laboratory findings is crucial when discussing the indication for resection or surveillance.

In this chapter, several clinical cases are presented to illustrate the typical features of the entities.

Serous Cystic Neoplasm (SCN) - Microcystic Adenoma

Serous cystic neoplasms comprise serous microcystic adenomas, serous oligocystic adenomas and the very rare serous cystadenocarcinoma. They are mostly located in the pancreatic body and tail, and do not show a connection to the pancreatic duct.

This 61 year old female patient was diagnosed with a cystic pancreatic tumor when she had an abdominal CT-scan for acute sigmoid diverticulitis.

For further differentiation of the cystic tumor, an MRI was performed (Figure 1).

In this patient, typically, the small cysts are separated by thin septae and grouped around a central scar that sometime shows calcifications. As the patient had lost two close relatives due to a pancreatic ductal adenocarcinoma, she insisted on surgical resection.

After laparotomy and opening of the omental pouch, the cystic tumor was seen in the proximal pancreatic corpus (Figure 2).

The pancreatic segment with the tumor was mobilized and a central pancreatic segment resection was performed (Figure 3).

The surgical specimen was centrally cut (Figure 4). The cystic tumor consists of many small cysts, pathognomonic for a serous microcystic adenoma.

A malignant transformation to a serous cystadenocarcinoma is very rare. Therefore, observation is the treatment of choice.

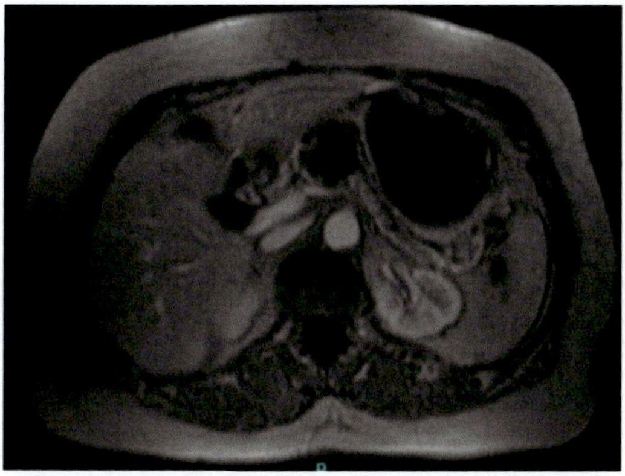

Figure 1. SCN MRI in a 61-year-old female patient.

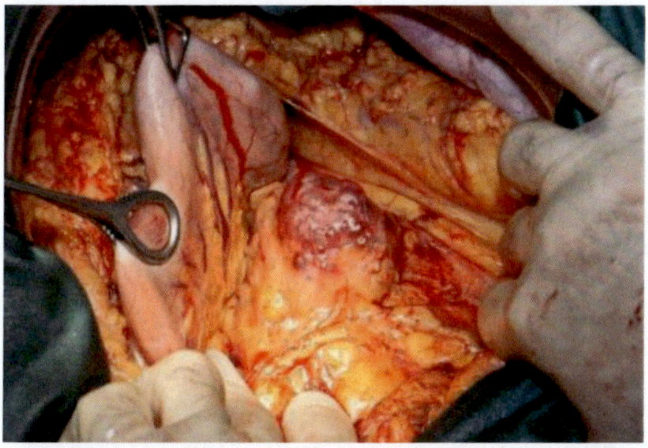

Figure 2. Cystic tumor in the central pancreas.

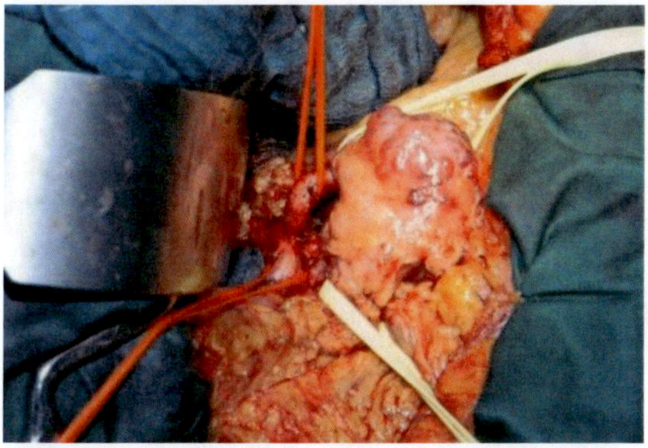

Figure 3. Mobilization of the pancreatic segment with the cystic tumor.

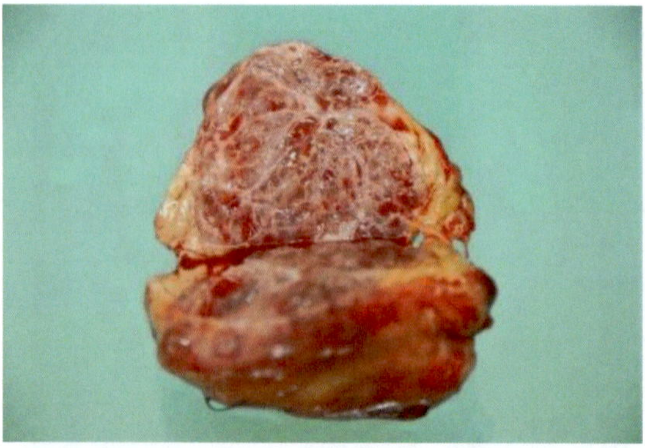

Figure 4. Transection of the surgical specimen typically shows multiple small cysts and a central scar.

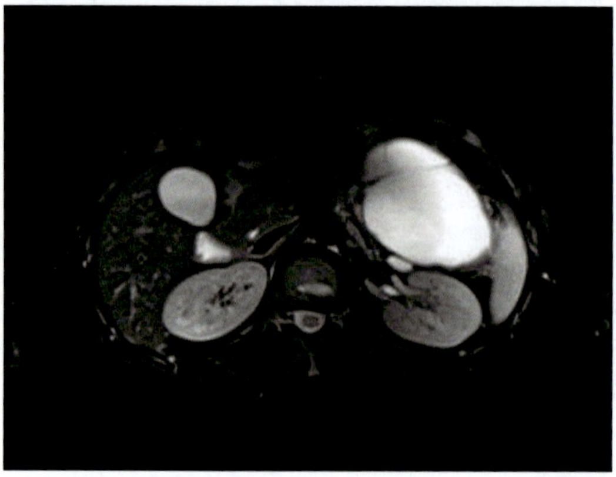

Figure 5. The MRI scan shows a large cystic tumor at the pancreatic tail with septae.

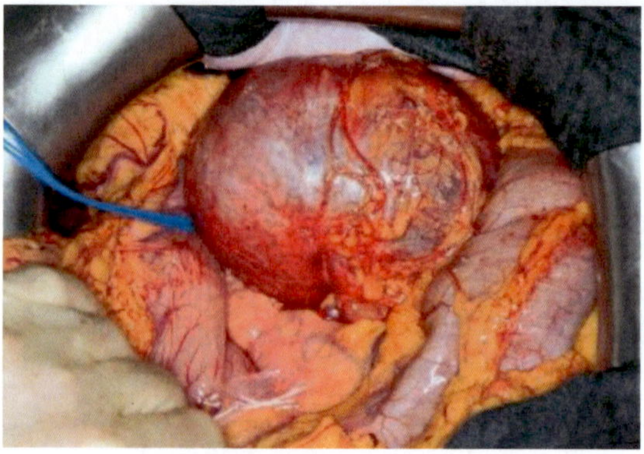

Figure 6. Large cyst in the left upper abdomen (oligocystic SCN).

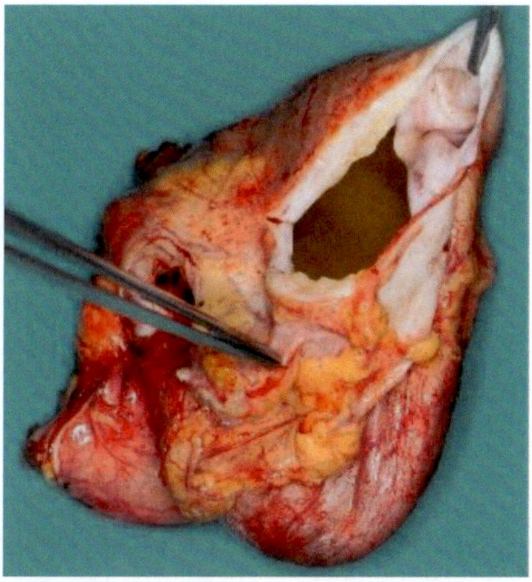

Figure 7. Surgical specimen of a SCN. The cyst is opened, the content is serous fluid.

Serous Cystic Neoplasm (SCN) - Oligocystic Adenoma

Serous oligocystic adenomas represent only 7-10% of all serous cystic neoplasias and consist of singular oder few larger cysts. Normally, they do not show a central scar or calcifications, but show the same histological features as serous microcystic forms [1-3].

The following, 65 year old, female patient presented with a growing mass in the upper left abdomen. The MRI scan show a cystic tumor in the pancreatic tail adjacent to the spleen with multiple septae (Figure 5). Neither connection to the pancreatic duct nor mural abnormalities were seen. Due to the growing discomfort, the patient decided for resection of the cystic tumor. Upon laparotomy, the cystic structure was easily found in the pancreatic tail (Figure 6).

A pancreatic tail resection was performed and later the specimen opened (Figure 7). The content of the large cyst was mainly serous fluid. Three slightly smaller cysts were separated by thin walls. Histology confirmed a serous cystadenoma and the postoperative course was uneventful.

Mucinous Cystic Neoplasm

The following patient was referred to us with a cystic tumor of the pancreatic tail. The female patient is 41 year old and the cyst was discovered upon sonography due to growing discomfort in the upper abdomen.

In a CT scan, a large cyst of the pancreatic tail is seen, no communication to the duct, no suspicious features of the cysts wall (Figure 8).

Initially, the cyst was interpreted as an pancreatic pseudocyst and endosonography was performed to discuss endosonographic drainage into the stomach. In the endosonographic puncture, however, mucinous fluid was aspirated and the patient sent for reevaluation. Due to the potential malignant potential of mucinous cystic tumors we decided for surgery [4, 5, 6].

Surgery was performed as a pancreatic tail resection including the spleen which was closely attached to the tumor. Intraoperatively, the typical round cyst with a fibrous pseudo capsule was seen (Figure 9).

When opening the specimen, viscous fluid and necrotic material could be extracted from the thick-walled cyst (Figure 10).

Mucinous cystic neoplasms of the pancreas almost exclusively arise in perimenopausal women, as in our case. Often, histologically an ovary like stroma is seen [7]. The wall often is considerably thicker than in serous neoplasms. Trabeculae can be seen and the cysts are lined with a mucin producing epithelium. Most of MCNs grow in the body and tail of the pancreas- as in our patient. Mural nodules can be early signs of malignant transformation [4].

Intraductal Papillary Neoplasm (IPMN)

Before 1996, all mucin producing tumors were summarized as mucinous cystic neoplasms (MCN) and only since then IPMN are seen as a distinct entity.

The following male, 67 years old patient presented with a history of three years of several episodes of upper abdominal, belt-shaped pain radiating into the back.

Clinical imaging showed a cystic tumor of the pancreatic head with a considerably enlarged pancreatic duct, suggestive for a main duct IPMN (Figure 11).

IPMNs are distinguished between main duct, side branch and mixed type IPMNs. In main duct IPMNs often the entire pancreatic duct is dilated by obstructing mucus and there for can mimic the symptoms of chronic pancreatitis as in our patient.

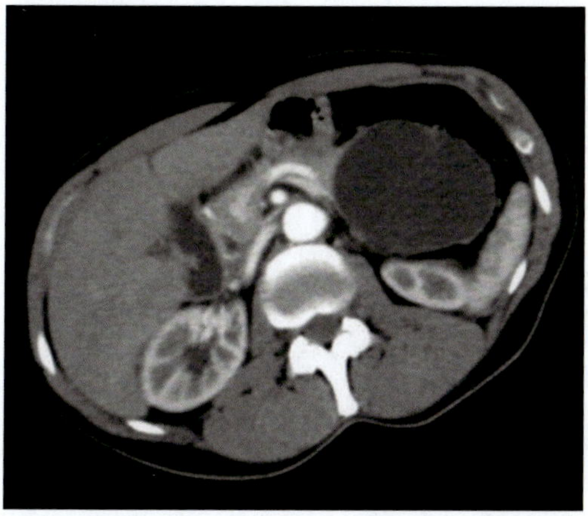

Figure 8. Cystic structure in the pancreatic tail, no septae, no communication to the pancreatic duct. (MCN).

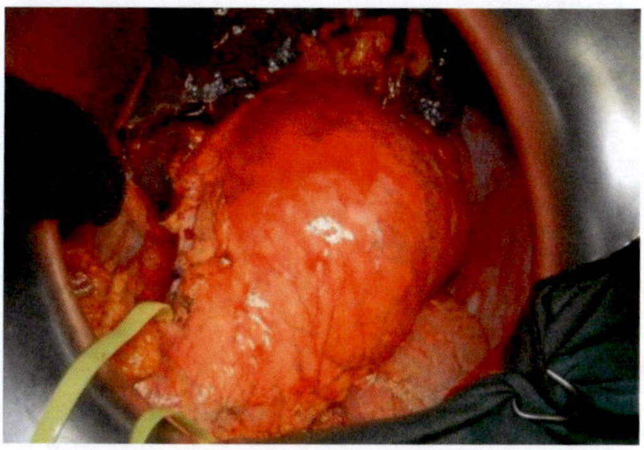

Figure 9. Cystic, well defined tumor of the pancreatic tail (MCN).

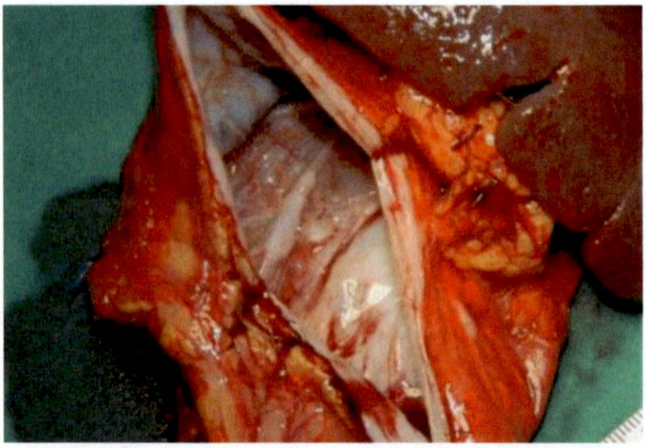

Figure 10. The opened specimen. A large amount of viscous fluid has been evacuated.

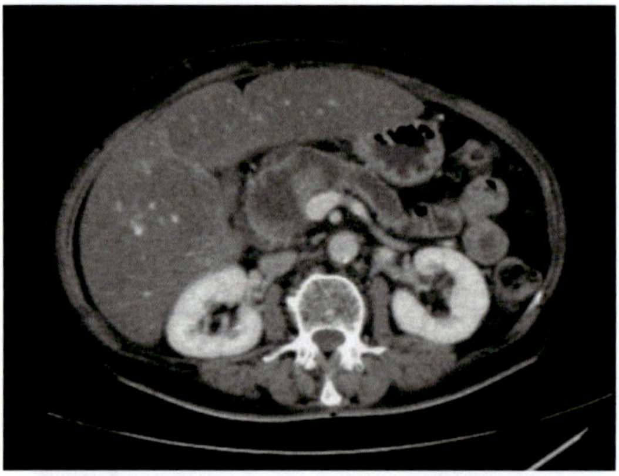

Figure 11. Cystic tumor of the pancreatic head with enlarged pancreatic duct (IPMN).

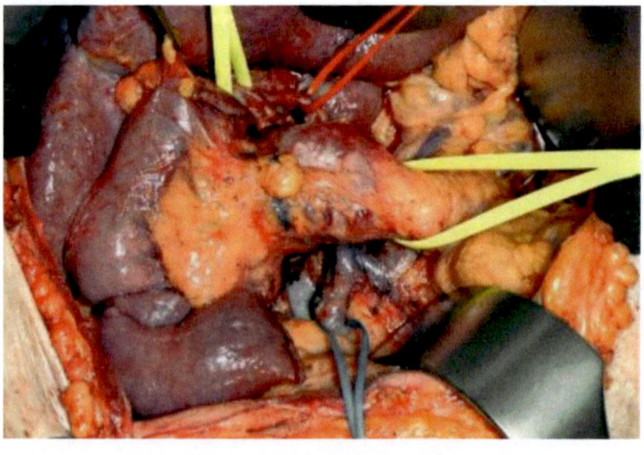

Figure 12. IPMN located between pancreatic head and corpus.

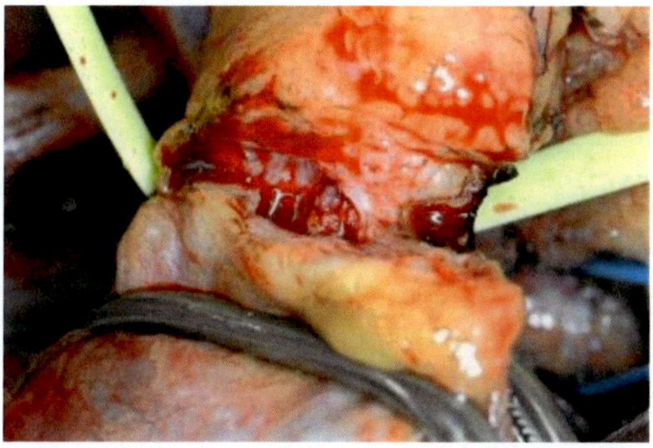

Figure 13. Papillary formations in the main pancreatic duct at transection.

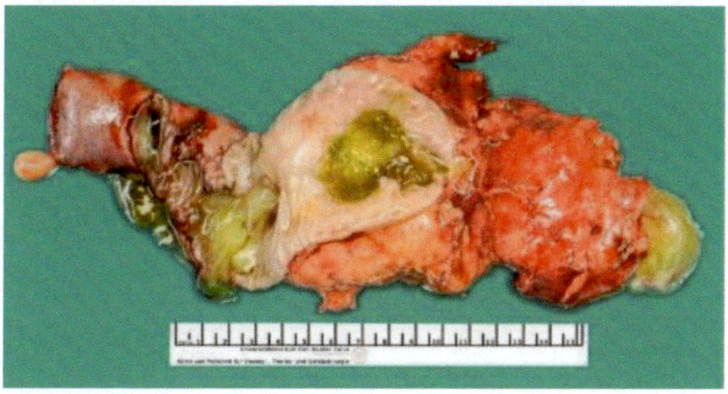

Figure 14. Surgical specimen of a main duct IPMN with obstructive mucus within the dilated duct.

Since main duct IPMNs have a considerable risk of malignant transformation [8, 9], we recommended the patient to undergo surgery. The tumor was located between pancreatic head and body (Figure 12) and the patient underwent pylorus preserving pancreatic head resection.

Upon transection of the pancreas, papillary formations were still found in pancreatic main duct that extended further two centimeters towards the pancreatic tail. (Figure 13) The pancreatic body was further mobilized and transected more distally until a free margin was reached.

Final pathologic evaluation of the specimen showed mucinous masses in the dilated duct (Figure 14) and histologically a main duct IPMN with severe dysplasia.

The reconstruction during surgery was easy due to the dilatation of the duct and the fibrous transformation of the pancreatic tissue and the postoperative course uncomplicated. Some IPMNs grow multifocally and can arise metachronously in the pancreatic remnant. Therefore, lifelong surveillance is recommended. Interestingly, in patients with IPMNs there is a high prevalence of extrapancreatic malignomas such as gastric or colorectal cancers [10].

Solid Pseudopapillary Neoplasm (SPN)

Solid pseudopapillary neoplasms (SPN) almost exclusively occur in young women around 25 – 39 years and sometimes in children. [11] Upon diagnosis, SPNs often are already large (9-12cm) and their symptoms result from the displacement by their large size. Mostly, SPNs are soft and therefore do not lead to dilatation of the pancreatic duct or choledochus. This was also the case in the slim 26 year old female patient who presented with a bulge in the upper left abdomen at her family practioner. MRI scan of the abdomen showed the large cystic mass with a solid peripheral part, cystic parts and hemorrhages which can help with the differential diagnosis in imaging (Figure 15).

Although the malignant potential of SPNs is considered to be low with around 15% [12], most SPNs are nevertheless resected due to their size and their displacing, space-consuming growth. Upon laparotomy, the large tumor was easily mobilized with the pancreatic tail and the adjacent spleen (Figure 16).

The surgical specimen typically showed degenerative necrotic changes with cavity formations (Figure 17).

Final histologic diagnosis revealed a SPN without malignant transformation and the postoperative course in the young patient was uneventful. No further treatment or surveillance is needed.

Cystic Degeneration of a Ductal Adenocarcinoma

The following patient presented with jaundice, pruritus and loss of weight and appetite in our medical department. Sonographically, an intra- and extrahepatic dilatation of the biliary tract was seen together with a tumor of the pancreatic head. In the CT-scan, a cystic tumor of the pancreatic head with partially solid formations was seen (Figure 18a). In a MRCP (Figure 18b), a pronounced dilatation of the pancreatic duct and multiple cysts in the head of the pancreas were seen.

The patient underwent pylorus-preserving pancreatoduodenectomy. Pathology showed a T3 N1 L0 V0 Pn1 R0 G2 ductal adenocarcinoma of the pancreas (PDAC) with intense desmoplasia (Figure 19).

Upon transection of the surgical specimen (Figure 20), the desmoplasia as well as the cystic degeneration of the massively dilated and coiled pancreatic duct could be seen. Most probably, the massive congestion due to the pronounced desmoplasia had led to a coiled dilatation of the pancreatic (and bile) duct that appeared like a cystic tumor of the pancreatic head.

Obviously, rarely even PDACs can mimic cystic tumors of the pancreas when the dilation of the ducts is accordingly pronounced. The occurrence of jaundice in a cystic tumor of the pancreas, however, should always raise the suspicion of malignancy [8].

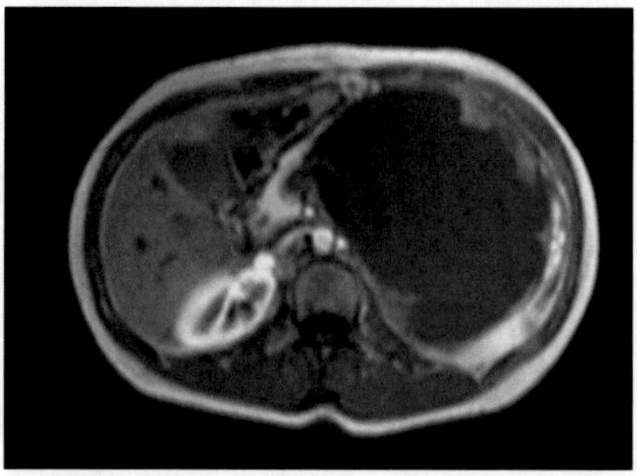

Figure 15. Typical large SPN with cystic and solid parts.

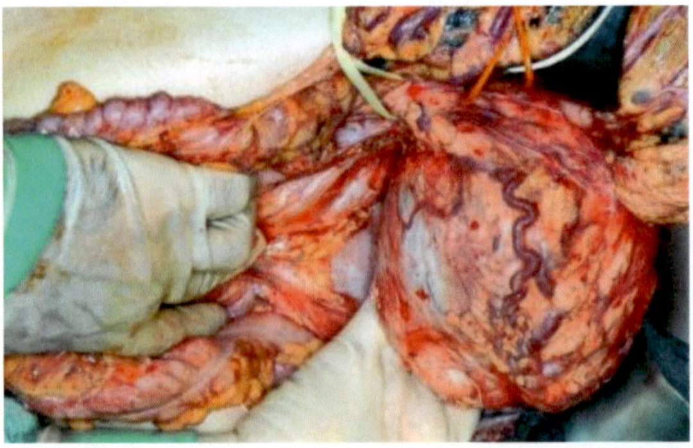

Figure 16. Large cystic tumor (SPN), well defined and mobile at the pancreatic tail.

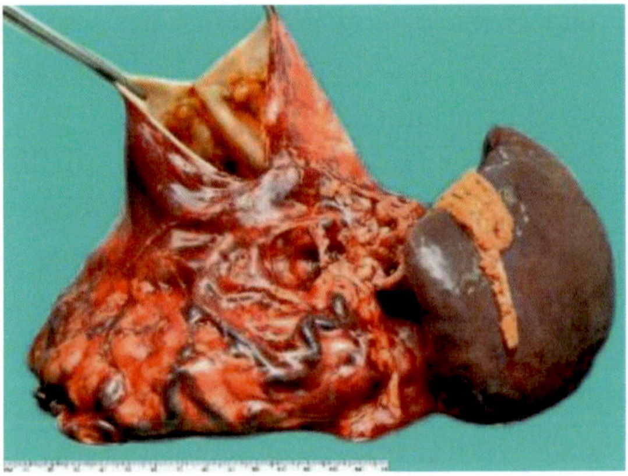

Figure 17. SPN with pancreatic tails and spleen, wall of the cyst opened and necrotic tissue removed.

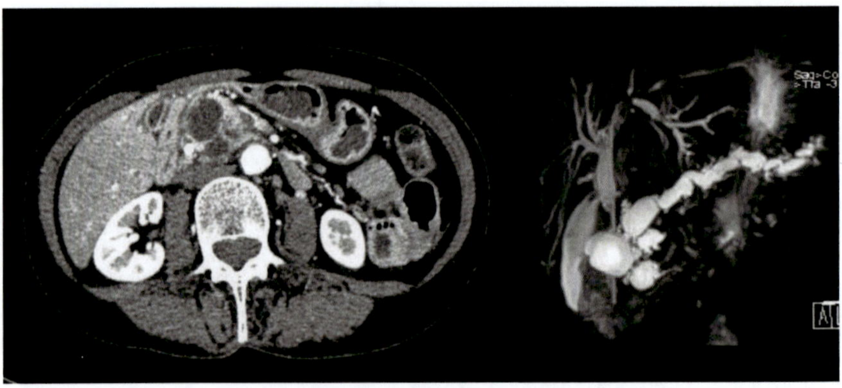

Figure 18. Cystic tumor of the pancreatic head in a) CT-scan and b) MRI.

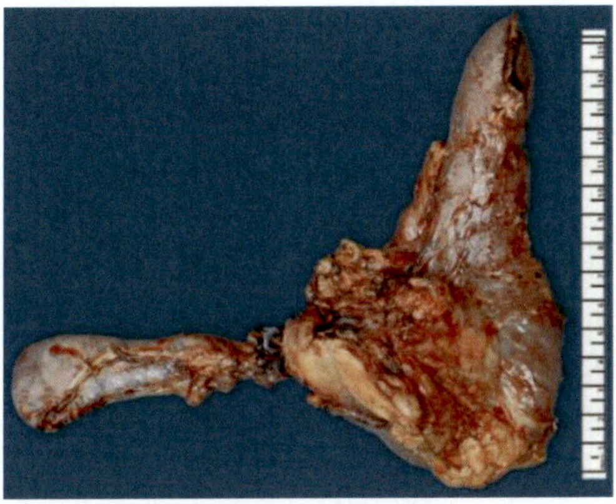

Figure 19. Pylorus-preserving pancreatoduodenectomy specimen, T3N1.

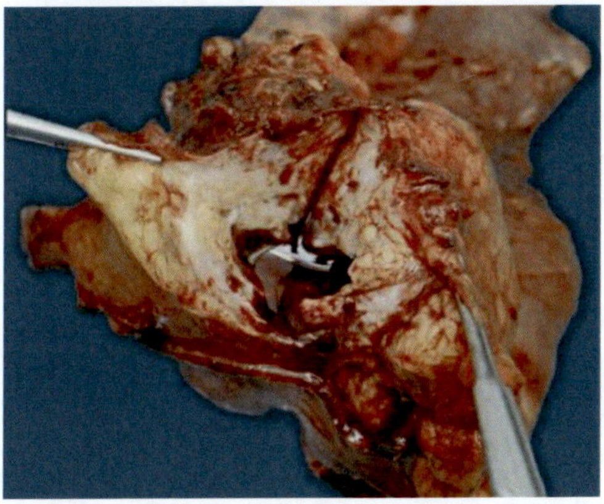

Figure 20. Cystic degeneration and dilatation of the pancreatic duct.

REFERENCES

[1] Cohen-Scali F, Vilgrain V, Brancatelli G et al. (2003) Discrimination of unilocular macrocystic serous cystadenoma from pancreatic pseudocyst and mucinous cystadenoma with CT: initial observations. *Radiology* 228: 727–733.

[2] Goh BKP, Tan YM, Yap WM etal. (2006) Pancreatic serous oligocystic adenomas: clinicopathologic features and a comparison

with serous microcystic adenomas and mucinous cystic neoplasms. *World J Surg* 30: 1553–1559.

[3] Khurana B, Mortelé KJ, Glickman J et al. (2003) Macrocystic serous adenoma of the pancreas: radiologic pathologic correlation. *AJR* 181: 119–123.

[4] Crippa S, Salvia R, Warshaw AL, Dominguez I, Bassi C, Falconi M, et al. Mucinous cystic neoplasm of the pancreas is not an aggressive entity: lessons from 163 resected patients. *Annals of surgery.* 2008;247(4):571-9.

[5] Zamboni G, Scarpa A, Bogina G, Iacono C, Bassi C, Talamini G, et al. Mucinous cystic tumors of the pancreas: clinicopathological features, prognosis, and relationship to other mucinous cystic tumors. *The American journal of surgical pathology.* 1999;23(4):410-22.

[6] Del Chiaro M, Verbeke C, Salvia R, Kloppel G, Werner J, McKay C, et al. European experts' consensus statement on cystic tumours of the pancreas. *Digestive and liver disease: official journal of the Italian Society of Gastroenterology and the Italian Association for the Study of the Liver.* 2013;45(9):703-11.

[7] Zamboni G, Scarpa A, Bogina G et al. (1999) Mucinous cystic tumors of the pancreas: clinicopathological features, prognosis, and relationship to other mucinous cystic tumors. *Am J Surg Pathol* 23: 410– 422.

[8] Grützmann R, Saeger HD. [Cystic tumors of the pancreas]. *Der Chirurg; Zeitschrift fur alle Gebiete der operativen Medizin.* 2010;81(8):755-68.

[9] Tanaka M, Chari S, Adsay V, Fernandez-del Castillo C, Falconi M, Shimizu M, et al. International consensus guidelines for management of intraductal papillary mucinous neoplasms and mucinous cystic neoplasms of the pancreas. *Pancreatology: official journal of the International Association of Pancreatology.* 2006;6(1-2):17-32.

[10] Christensen JA, Fletcher JG, Fidler JL et al. (2004) Intraductal papillary mucinous neoplasms of the pancreas: CT patterns of recurrence and multiob- server performance in detecting recurrent neoplasms. *AJR* 183: 1367–1374.

[11] Cantisani V, Mortele KJ, Levy A et al. (2003) MR imaging features of solid pseudopapillary tumor of the pancreas in adult and pediatric patients. *AJR* 181: 395–401.

[12] Tipton SG, Smyrk TC, Sarr MG, Thompson GB. Malignant potential of solid pseudopapillary neoplasm of the pancreas. *The British journal of surgery*. 2006;93(6):733-7.

About the Editor

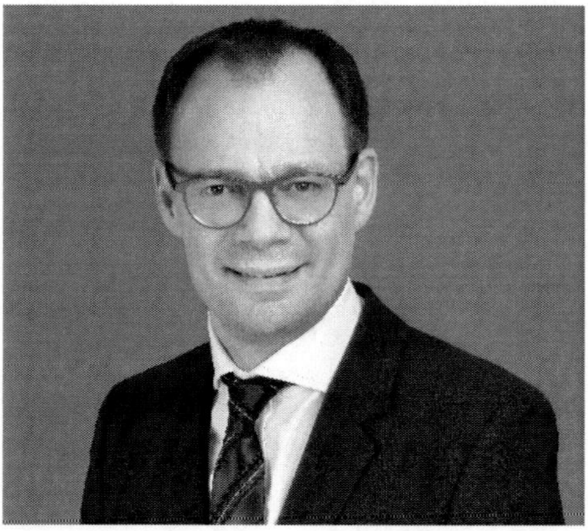

Robert Grützmann, MD, PhD, MBA
Professor of Surgery, Head of the Department,
Department of Surgery,
Director of the Surgical Department,
University Hospital Erlangen, Germany
University Nuremberg-Erlangen, Germany

Before becoming head of the surgical department of the university hospital of the Friedrich-Alexander-University of Erlangen-Nuremberg in October 2015, Prof. Dr. med. Robert Grützmann, MBA, specialist for general surgery, Hepato-Pancreato-Biliary-(HPB) surgery and vascular surgery was working among other things as director of the PancreasCenter of the University Hospital Dresden. He completed his medical studies from 1990 to 1997 at the Charité in Berlin. Afterwards, he worked for a few months at the Boston Consulting Group (BCG), largest company consultancy, then at the University Hospital Dresden, where he acquired three specialisations and the "Master of Business Administration in Health Care Management". He finished his PhD in 2005 on "The molecular biology characterization and validation of candidate genes in sporadic and familial Pancreatic carcinoma" becoming in the process an international specialist for pancreatic cancer. He achieved numerous prizes, such as the von-Langenbeck Prize of the Germans Society of Surgery. Further milestones of his professional carieer were in Dresden becoming Senior Chief Physician at the Clinic and Polyclinic for Visceral, Thoracic and Vascular Surgery in 2012, Deputy Director of the "University Vascular Center" in 2013, and Director of the The pancreas cancer center of the University Cancer Center Dresden in 2014.

INDEX

D

E

F

G

H

I

K

L

M

N

O

P

R

S

T

U

V

W